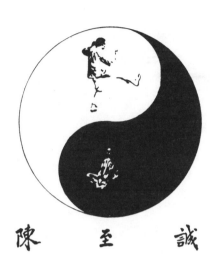

陳　至　誠

太極拳力學和自衛

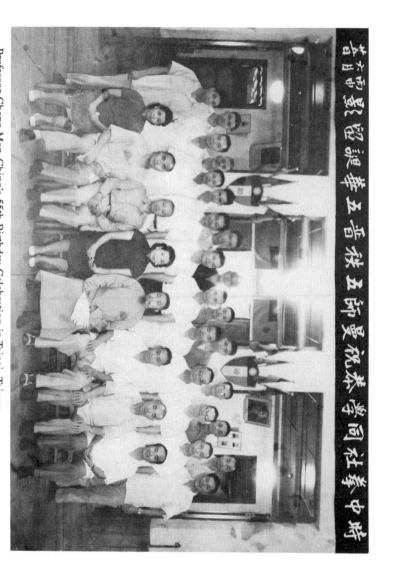

華封三祝五福五常壽五百壽五師畏德求學同社畫史中州

六五南熙切親日即

Professor Cheng Man-Ching's 55th Birthday Celebration in Taipei, Taiwan

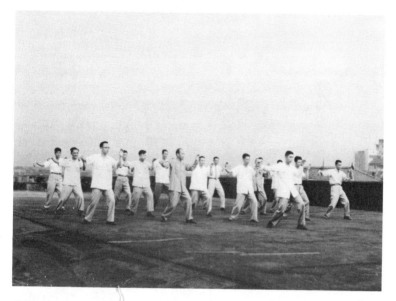

William C.C. Chen's Tai Chi Chuan class of the Postal and
Telecommunication Bureau of Taipei, Taiwan 1950's

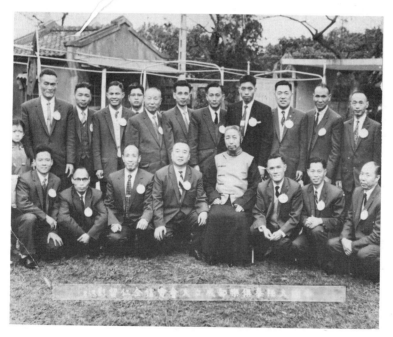

William C.C. Chen and the Tai Chi Chuan members of the Postal and
Telecommunications Bureau, taken with Professor Cheng Man-Ching in
Taipei, Taiwan 1950's

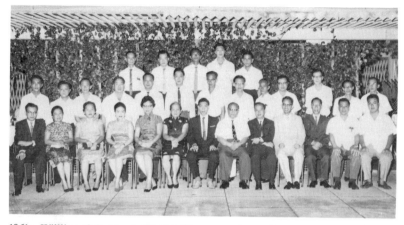

1961—Willliam C.C. Chen's Tai Chi Chuan members—Singapore

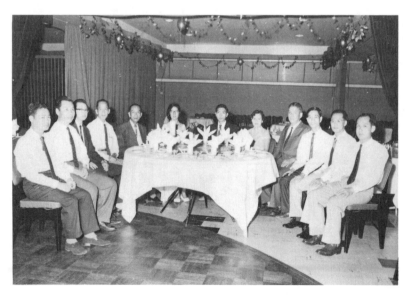

1961—William C.C. Chen's Tai Chi Chuan members—Kuala Lumpur, Malaysia

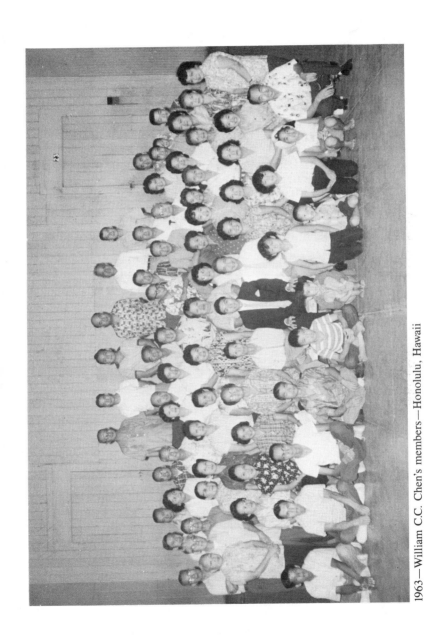

1963—William C.C. Chen's members—Honolulu, Hawaii

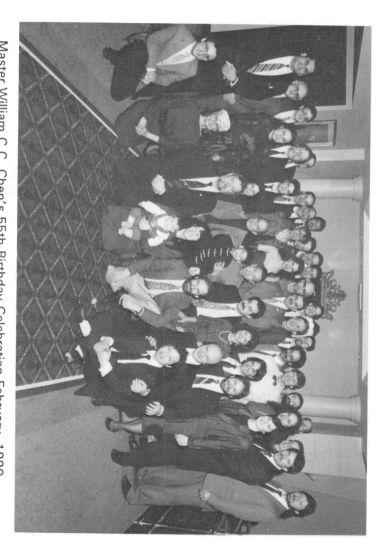

Master William C.C. Chen's 55th Birthday Celebration February, 1990

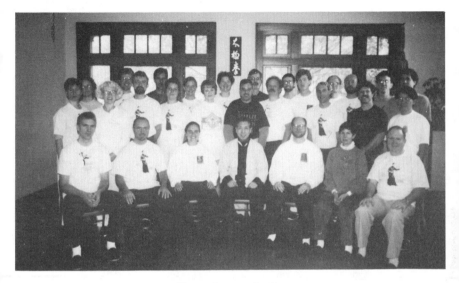

Bloomington Indiana
Tai Chi Chuan Association of Indiana

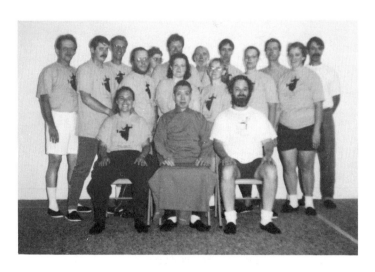

Davenport Iowa
Laura Stone & Scott Caulpetzer

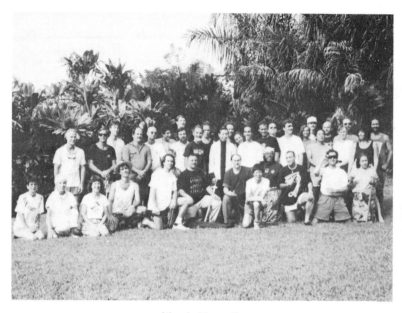

Maui, Hawaii
Hawaii Tai Chi Chuan Association

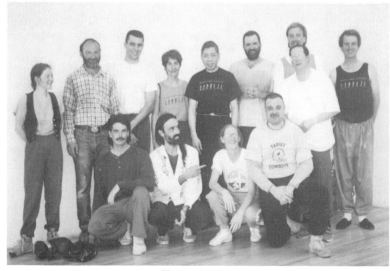

Tucson, Arizona
Jeffery Zauderer

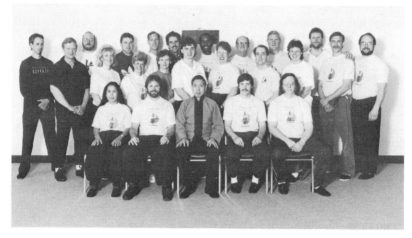

Erie, Pennsylvania
Body Awareness

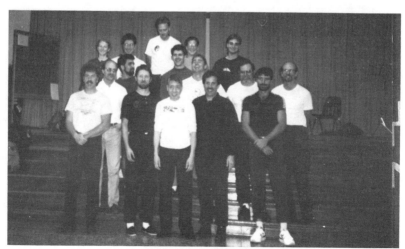

Baltimore, Maryland
Mark K. Bayne

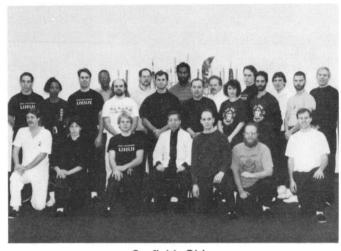

Garfield, Ohio
International Kung Fu Center

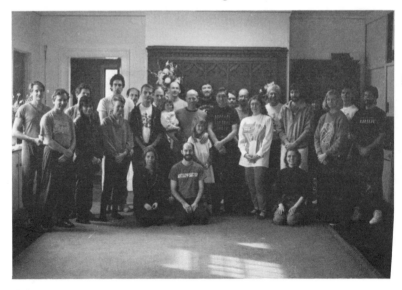

Newton, Massachusetts
Alan Shapiro

Contents

ACKNOWLEDGEMENTS

Special acknowledgement must be given to my wife, Priscilla S. Chen. This book would not have been possible without her support, encouragement and cooperation.

In 1982, Valentin Chu suggested that I write the text of this book. I am grateful for his time and help. I also sincerely thank the following people, whose time and energy helped make this book possible.

James Moore and
Winston Chin . . . . . . Photo of The Movements

Anthony Manderino . . . . Cover Photo
Scott Rodell . . . . Cover Design
John Amira . . . . Arrows on photographs

Gary Benson . . . . Typesetting

Timothy Pitt
Louis Shapiro
Rolly Brown
Linda Lehrhaupt . . . . Editing

George Blank
Norman Blair
Ken Lipson
Carol Mancuso
Eric Weitzner . . . . Proofreading

William C.C. Chen

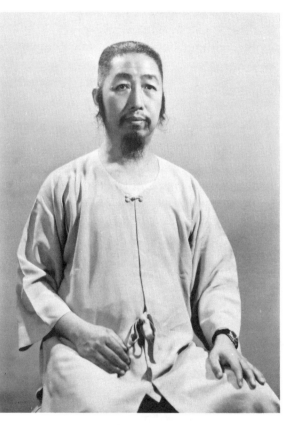

至誠賢弟存念

庚子鄭曼髯

Professor Chen Man-Ching
World-Renowned Grandmaster of Tai Chi Chuan
This autographed photo was presented to me
from my teacher in 1960.

Published by
William C. C. Chen
2 Washington Square Village #10J
New York,   NY 10012
phone: 212   675-2816
   fax: 212   677-5352

website: WILLIAMCCCHEN.COM
   email: WmCCChen@aol.com

4th printing 1989
5th printing 1992
6th printing 1994
7th printing 1997
8th printing 1999

Printed in the United States of America

What is Tai Chi Chuan

Tai Chi Chuan, literally meaning "the Grand Ultimate Fist," is one of the most sophisticated Chinese martial arts. Originally Tai Chi Chuan was vigorous as well as gentle, containing rigid-soft and rapid-slow movements, with total body coordination and great mental control. During actual fighting, a master of Tai Chi Chuan could make his body as soft as cotton, but at the instant of delivering the punch, suddenly become as hard as steel. One moment he was as motionless as a mountain, the next as swift as ocean tides. Achieving such unpredictable, alternate changes of dynamics can lead to the highest level of martial tactics, whether in competitions among masters or for self-defense against muggers and similar street attackers.

These interactions of soft-hard tactics, as those of Yin-Yang, are all based on a well-known concept of Chinese philosophy as propounded in the *I Ching* (Book of Changes). Therefore, the symbol of Yin-Yang and the name of Tai Chi were adopted for this particular martial art. In the old days, it was kept as a precious secret, taught only to a few chosen disciples who were both physically strong and morally sound.

The graceful, slow-flowing style of the present-day Tai Chi Chuan, coupled with a complete relaxation of the body and mind, did not appear until the 1930's. It took three generations for the famous Yang family to modify it. This unique and beneficial innovation made Tai Chi Chuan suitable for all: young or old, male or female, strong or weak. It incurs no risk, involves no equipment, and requires very little space for maneuvering. Hence the number of Tai Chi Chuan practitioners has increased tremendously. Today, millions are practicing it daily in China, Southeast Asia, Europe, and the Americas. It is not inconceivable that someday there may be billions of people practicing this ancient martial art.

At present, Tai Chi Chuan is known as both a Chinese martial art and a calisthenic. In the heat of fighting, most martial artists find it difficult to keep calm and loose. The slow and even movements of Tai Chi Chuan tend to relax the body and mind, promoting the flow of vital energy (chi) and replacing stiffness with flexibility and good body coordination. This helps fighters to effectively reach the highest level in the art of self-defense. Practiced daily and properly as an exercise, it promotes one's mental tranquility, improves physical fitness, increases blood circulation to its full capacity, and provides the tissues of the various organs with the maximum amount of oxygen. It also prevents or even cures certain forms of sickness, such as arthritis, rheumatism, and hypertension. Tai Chi Chuan is really a priceless treasure.

An Internal System

All the movements of Tai Chi Chuan are activated by pressure changes in the lower abdomen. As the pressure increases, the arms flow outward or upward. When it decreases the arms move inward or downward. The arms never move by themselves without the abdominal pressure changes. Chinese Tai Chi Chuan players often say: (太 極 拳 不 動 手 . 動 手 非 太 極 拳) which means that, in the movements of Tai Chi Chuan the arms never move alone or independently. If they do, the movements are not considered as Tai Chi Chuan.

Abdominal pressure is the main source of power, especially, the center point of the lower abdomen, known as "Tan Tien" (丹 田). "Tan Tien" literally translates as "field of Cinnabar," which means it is a very important point. When we practice Tai Chi Chuan, we should place our mind in the lower abdominal area, and let mind, body and energy act as one unit, since all the motions of Tai Chi Chuan are created by the energy force from inside the body, rather than from the outside. That is why Tai Chi Chuan is an internal system of martial art.

Characteristics

This Chinese martial art is the best known of the internal systems. It emphasizes body coordination and inner energy (Chi), rather than muscle power, which is considered secondary. The mental concentration, deep breathing, relaxing and sinking of the body, plus body weight shifting and pressing, generate a tremendous inner energy flow throughout the system, resulting in the movements of Tai Chi Chuan.

The slow, soft and gentle Tai Chi Chuan movements are like waves of the ocean. They push and merge into one another, creating a continuous flow of energy, seemingly with no beginning and no end. These gentle movements, combined with a relaxation of the body and the mind, are sometimes called "meditation in motion."

Practicing the movements is the same as being in an imaginary fight with several opponents. This combat training, done in slow motion in the same manner as a beginner practices typing, helps loosen tense muscles and joints, promoting automatic body alignment and a solid center of gravity. It develops good body coordination, eliminating mistakes and bad habits. This results in the conservation of energy and gets the job done well. It is also an excellent way of working out for Western-style boxers and for practitioners of any other style of martial arts, both as preparation before facing a serious match and as daily training.

The slow motion of Tai Chi Chuan mainly attracts more intellectual and mature people, because one needs to see deeply in order to understand its basic principle and go beyond the comparatively simple punches and kicks powered solely by muscle strength. By staying calm and relaxed, you are able to size up and deal with any situation as it arises. Male or female, old or young, weak or strong, you will definitely receive great benefits by regularly and faithfully practicing Tai Chi Chuan, whether for physical health, mental well-being, or for the art of self-defense—even just for the joy of life.

Speed

The full capacity of speed for punches and kicks can be achieved through the practice of the slow and soft movements of Tai Chi Chuan. The nature of the slow motion or quick action from the human body is created by pressure changes within the body. Small pressure changes that gradually increase or decrease create the slow, soft and gentle movements of Yang Style Tai Chi Chuan. Greater pressure and more rapid increases produce faster motion. The force of a technique, such as a punch, push or kick, depends upon the speed and magnitude of the pressure change. An example of this principle is a bullet rushing out from a fired gun. The muzzle velocity of a bullet depends on the degree of explosive power within the cartridge. More explosive power, the greater the change in pressure. The result: greater speed and more impact power.

According to the Remington Center Fire Rifle Cartridges ballistics' table, published in Robert A. Scanlon's *Law Enforcement Bible* in 1978:

The Springfield 30-06C bullet, with a weight of 125 grains, has a muzzle velocity of 3140 feet per second. At 500 yards, the velocity is 1600 feet per second with an impact force of 705 foot pounds.

The Winchester 30-30C bullet, which also has a weight of 125 grains, has a muzzle velocity of 2570 feet per second. At 500 yards, the velocity is 960 feet per second with an impact force of 260 foot pounds.

Both bullets have the same weight (125 grains*), yet at 500 yards the 30-06C bullet is more than one and a half times faster than the 30-30C bullet with almost three times the impact force. The difference lies in the cartridges. The 30-06C cartridge is longer and a little wider, and contains more gunpowder. It produces more explosive power and generates more force when fired.

Type of Bullet Federal Load No.	Bullet Wgt. in Grains	Velocity (Feet per Second)		Energy (Foot Pound) 500 Yds
		Muzzle	500 Yds	
Springfield 30-06C	125	3140	1600	705
Winchester 30-30C	125	2570	960	260

*The Measurements of the cartridges are derived from *Cartridges of The World*, 5th Edition © 1985 By Frank C. Barnes Edited by Ken Warer

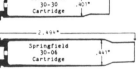

Another example of the same principle of pressure change is the rapid release of air pressure which results in the swift motion of a flying balloon. When a balloon is blown up to full size and then suddenly released, it flies away at a great speed. If the same balloon is blown up only half-way and then released, it flies away slowly. The speed depends on air pressure changes within the balloon. In order to generate rapid punches, kicks and ducking or neutralizing movements, one must be able to change tension from very relaxed to very tense within a split second or vice versa.

The primary requirement for self-defense is that punches and kicks must be delivered with maximum force, and force depends on speed. Speed is the main source of power. In physics, speed is the most indispensable element of power. If you double the mass, the power only doubles; but if you double the speed you have four times the power. A punch or kick without speed is the same as a motionless bullet: powerless and useless. It is naturally easier to be tense than to be loose before or during a punch or kick. It is also very difficult to stay loose while being punched or kicked. The essence of Tai Chi Chuan is to remain calm and loose. This allows the full range of tension changes, and the maximum speed for any action.

The great champion heavyweight boxer of the 1920's, Jack "The Giant Killer" Dempsey, referred to his powerful punches as a body explosion. That meant he was able to keep his body relaxed until the punch was delivered, putting his whole body in motion, like an exploding bomb. His punches were generated by enormous and instantaneous tension changes. Therefore, we often see good martial artists or boxers in the ring who are able to control their body tension to stay loose and relaxed for any fast action, and do not rely only on strong arm muscles for delivering powerful blows.

The speed of punches, pushes, kicks, or neutralization of an opponent's attack depends on the degree of the tension change, either from no tension to very tense or from very tense to very loose. Any dynamic motion must be created by the interchange of two opposite forces, from positive to negative, loose to tense, Yin and Yang, or vice versa. Thus, for the art of self-defense, there is neither absolute forcefulness, nor absolute softness. Martial artists who practice a hard style should take the opportunity to participate in a Tai Chi Chuan program. Learning to stay more relaxed would enable them to increase speed for any necessary action. On the other hand, Tai Chi Chuan practitioners who are able to maintain body relaxation, should not overlook tension training, in order to fulfill the fundamental Taoist's Tai Chi principle of Yin and Yang.

Speed Progress Chart

The following chart shows, in simplified form, the progress of increasing the speed of punches and kicks that results from the study of Tai Chi Chuan versus a hard-style martial art. According to my principles, the human body's actions are generated by changes in tension within the body; the greater the degree of change in tension, the greater the speed.

Thus, my theory is that there are two basic ways to increase the speed of punches and kicks: 1) by increasing (maximizing) tension at the moment of impact, 2) by decreasing (minimizing) tension before the action occurs. The hard-style student progressively raises his maximum tension, while the Tai Chi Chuan student lowers his minimum tension.

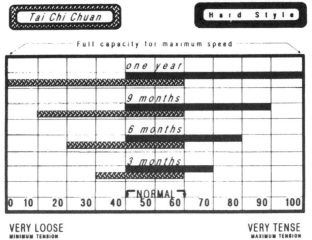

Up to a certain point, each will increase the speed of his punches and kicks at about the same rate. In order to achieve the maximum speed, however, the Tai Chi Chuan student must find a way to increase impact tension, the hard-style student will have to reduce his tension before the action takes place.

The chart shows that a person with no martial arts background, when preparing to strike, tenses his muscles to 40% of his potential. As he further tenses his arm muscles to punch, the tension reaches a maximum of 60%. Thus the increase is 20% of overall capacity. Every three months the student, training in a hard-style school, will be able to increase the amount he can tense his muscles by an additional 10% of his overall potential. Within one year, this student should reach 100% of his tension capacity; thus the speed of his strikes has increased at a satisfactory rate.

A student of Tai Chi Chuan and a hard-style practitioner will increase the speed of punches and kicks at a similar rate. However, the Tai Chi Chuan player will increase speed by reducing the amount of basal tension held in the body by 10% every three months. The level of maximum tension will remain at 60% in the Tai Chi Chuan student, but the overall increase when striking will be the same as that of a hard-style fighter.

The Tai Chi Chuan player's soft, loose, elastic body is able to tense only the muscles needed, and then instantly releases them. A relaxed body has the added benefits of increased energy and alertness, because less of the body's energy is wasted in tensing muscles unnecessarily. A loose, calm body is also more sensitive to incoming stimuli. Yet developing maximum impact tension is also very important. We can't have one without the other. In order to deliver punches and kicks with maximum speed, we must possess both looseness and tension, soft and hard. This is encompassed in the symbol of Tai Chi Chuan, "Yin and Yang."

For Physical and Mental Health

The Chinese have known for many centuries that Tai Chi Chuan was excellent for a person's body and mind. On the physical side it facilitates digestion, promotes blood circulation, benefits the kidneys and enables the body to utilize large amounts of oxygen through deep and natural breathing.

A person who has faithfully practiced Tai Chi Chuan for a long time derives many physical benefits from it. His body weight is properly adjusted, whether he was originally overweight or underweight. His blood vessels become softer, helping him to avoid and often reverse high blood pressure or the hardening of the arteries. His skin is smooth and rosy. His muscles are flexible and elastic, but can stiffen with extraordinary strength if necessary, as in the case of self-defense.

Tai Chi Chuan is good for any individual, whether a muscular man or a slender woman, an active adolescent or a white-haired grand-mother. It does not strain the body with harsh movements, but tunes up its natural functions. It gives a person the best form of health and fitness.

The benefits of Tai Chi Chuan on the mind is as significant as on the body. From the moment we were born, we have possessed instinctive desires for food, comfort, affections and other pleasures. These desires grow stronger and multiply as the baby becomes a child, and the child becomes an adult. They could be endless in the pursuit of our goals in friendship, love, marriage, wealth and success, or just merely of a chance to survive in famine or war.

This is true whether we live in an underdeveloped land or a technologically advanced country, whether we are rich or poor, beautiful or ugly, successful or otherwise. The problems may be different, but their effect on us are the same. We suffer from frustrations and tensions in various degrees, resulting in what the psychologists call "stress," which is harmful to both the body and the mind.

As a health tonic, Tai Chi Chuan can make us physically and mentally sound. Its slow and gentle movements act to "lubricate" every part of the body and relax the mind. This ancient system renders our thinking lucid, turns our temper gentle and brings us peace of mind that helps us to function well in our hectic modern world—whether in education, career or social relations. It enables a person to reach the goal of what the ancient Chinese sages called "the golden mean," in which human desires and frustrations are effectively harnessed for the ultimate benefit of the individual.

It is no wonder that many thousands of people in the United States have found Tai Chi Chuan a sound exercise for the body as well as an effective spiritual preparation for facing everyday problems.

Breathing

Proper breathing plays a primary role in the movements of Tai Chi Chuan. This is controlled by contracting and releasing the diaphragm. The oxygen taken in from the air supports the immediate needs of billions of body cells and removes carbon dioxide from the blood. This is essential to our life. Going without water or food for days would not have fatal results, but even a few minutes without oxygen would result in brain damage or death.

Tai Chi Chuan is based on the natural way of breathing: it is slow, gentle and deep. Natural breathing increases lung capacity, supplies sufficient oxygen for the body's needs and aids in relaxation during the movements. It also helps to loosen all passages, allowing the distribution of oxygen more effectively and evenly. During inhalation, the diaphragm goes down, which increases the size of the lung cavity and forces more air to rush in. Exhaling moves the diaphragm up and squeezes the waste air out. This mechanical motion is comparable to that of a bellows.

Inhaled and exhaled air passes through the natural hair filters of the nose. The mouth should be kept closed, which prevents it from becoming dry. In fighting, keeping the mouth closed will help avoid biting the tongue, breaking the jaw and becoming exhausted. Initiate the breath with the diaphragm, not the nose. Otherwise, the benefits of natural breathing will be reduced. When the breath is initiated with the nose, only the upper part of the lungs are filled with air; the chest will become tense, causing the body to lose its center of gravity. Breathing in this manner is normally short, unhealthy and sometimes a sign of illness.

In the process of doing Tai Chi Chuan slowly, the movements are soft, gentle and flow continuously. The mind and body are relaxed, the breathing is long, deep and very calm. While inhalation is taking place, the diaphragm is contracted down to the lower abdomen, abdominal pressure is increased and the energy begins to flow. At this time, the arms are moving outward or upward. During exhalation, the diaphragm is released, abdominal pressure is decreased and the flow of energy subsides. Now, the arms are moving inward or downward.

Once the mind, body and energy are unified, natural breathing will take place. This will result in full energy flow for the movements, and creates a perfect motion of soft pushes, punches and kicks.

In sparring, fighting or lifting weights, the breathing is different than in the solo form of Tai Chi Chuan. In addition to the breathing, we must pay attention to a third state, called "compression". That is holding the diaphragm downward while the thigh muscles exert force upward. This pressurization of the abdomen(Tan Tien) supports the spine, and serves a connecting link between the root and the fist. This all happens at the brief moment of impact; there is no time for breathing in or out.

The power of the strikes depends upon the degree of this compression. The greater the compression in the lower abdomen, the greater the power made available for the strike.

The Development of Tai Chi Chuan

In ancient China, battles among families, clans and districts were waged for centuries. In this kind of warring society, martial arts were the sole means of survival and self-protection. In time, specific forms and styles were developed in various localities where these skills were practiced. As the Chinese society became more civilized, special schools were formed to teach and improve the various martial arts systems. These conditions gave rise to hundreds of highly sophisticated martial arts systems in China. In those days, unique fighting techniques were jealously guarded like military secrets by the clans and schools practicing them.

The development of the internal system of kung-fu known as Tai Chi Chuan is generally attributed to Cheng San Feng, a 13th-century man who lived during the Sung Dynasty in China. He taught his skill to only a few disciples, who in turn passed it on to limited numbers of specially chosen students. In those days Tai Chi Chuan was a treasured system practiced by only a privileged few. It was not until a couple of centuries later that some of the masters began to teach large numbers of students, resulting in Tai Chi Chuan becoming popular as the number of people interested in the art grew.

By the early 19th century, Tai Chi Chuan began to evolve into several major styles and many minor forms. Chen Cheng-hsing (18th–19th century) put his personal imprint on what he practiced and taught, known as *Chen style,* that consists of vigorous as well as gentle movements. Since Tai Chi Chuan was potentially a new weapon in a martial society, he kept the techniques a secret within the Chen family for generations. However, a stranger named Yang Lu-chan (1799–1872) was determined to learn Tai Chi Chuan. He gained admission to the Chen household by posing as a servant, and spied on clan members as they practiced. He was eventually caught, but the old master was so impressed by Yang's skill and devotion that he taught him formally.

Yang Lu-chan known as "The Unsurpassed Yang" for his unique fighting ability, brought Tai Chi Chuan to Peking and taught it to the Palace Officials and to his sons. Thereafter his two sons taught it openly to the public.

Yang Chin-pu (1883–1936) one of the best known Tai Chi Chuan masters, was Yang Lu-chan's grandson (son of his second son). He apparently fell into extreme dissipation in the big city and as punishment his father locked him in an empty room where he was allowed no visitors. Since he had nothing to do in his "prison" but practice Tai Chi Chuan, he emerged as an invincible master. As he got older and became more experienced, he evolved his own style of Tai Chi Chuan. Now known as *Yang style* Tai Chi Chuan, it is much softer, slower and gentler than those practiced by his predecessors. It has moderate postures and well knit, lithe movements.

Wu Chien-chuan (1870–1942) was a young martial arts practitioner who had intense interest in hard or external style kung-fu. As he grew older, he realized the importance of the softness in internal systems such as Tai Chi Chuan. To remove the stiffness from his hard-style kung-fu, he learned Tai Chi Chuan from his father, Wu Chuan-yack (1834–

1902), whose teacher was Yang Pan-huo, first son of Yang Lu-chan. Not long after learning it, Wu won a martial arts tournament in China after World War I. He then opened his own Tai Chi Chuan school to teach the art to the public. His style, now known as *Wu style,* placed emphasis on low stances and widespread arms, involving more tension than the Yang style.

Sun Lu-tang (1860–1930) was also an expert in Pa-Kua and Hsing-I. His style of Tai Chi Chuan, known as *Sun style,* with dexterous and nimble movements performed at a quick tempo and with lively footwork, was greatly influenced by the other two styles.

Among the Yang style masters was Professor Cheng Man-ching (1900–1975). He was one of the most talented artists of this era, with 5 accomplishments: poetry, painting, calligraphy, traditional Chinese medicine and Tai Chi Chuan. In his late twenties, he learned the full version long form 128 postures, from Grandmaster Yang Chin-pu, but had the intelligence and foresight to abridge it to a short form of 37 postures, so that it required less time and was easier to learn, while still giving the same benefits as the long form. This short form has gained great acceptance among practitioners all over the United States, Asia, and even Europe.

Today the Yang and Wu styles (mostly the short forms) are practiced widely in the Far East, America and Europe. The People's Republic of China has its own short form of 24 postures. Besides my 60 movements of Tai Chi Chuan, many of my former classmates and other Tai Chi Chuan experts in Hong Kong have also devised their own short forms.

There are now dozens, perhaps hundreds of varieties of short forms. They differ in the inclusion and exclusion of some of the repetitions of postures from the long form, without changing the principles and philosophy on which Tai Chi Chuan was based.

William C. C. Chen's 60 Movements

William C. C. Chen's 60 movements are derived from Prof. Cheng Man-ching's 37 Postures. I am using the term "movement," which I feel is more descriptive than that of "posture." The reason I have modified Prof. Cheng's short form is because during my first decade of teaching I was often asked by my students about the "missing parts" of the Yang-style form. It was not until I had gained 20 years of experience that I felt confident to make a change by adding on various parts and removing some repetitions.

The 60 movements I have now adapted remain the same in basic idea and principle. The length of the movements remains unchanged, but I count each individual posture and each repetition as a movement. All movements are as slow, soft and gentle in a continuous flow as the original Yang-style of Prof. Cheng's short form.

However, compared to versions generally taught, my 60 revolving movements are slightly higher in stance and smaller in step. This difference is intentional. In the slow motion of Tai Chi Chuan, much of the body weight is on a single leg. If the student is relaxed, as he should be, his weight tends to sink down. As a result, it may cause a certain fatigue and exhaustion in the legs which leads to an unconscious tensing of the upper body. Ultimately this might affect the smooth flow of inner energy and body coordination. My high stances and smaller steps are designed to prevent such a possibility.

Since I put great emphasis on Tai Chi Chuan as a superior form of martial art, I pay special attention to the smooth working of body coordination and energy flow, because they are the main source of power. Thus, in my class I often urge my students to "press down and bounce up," which means to sink one's energy into the leg and down to the foot, then to pump it up through the arms, palms and fists all the way into the fingers. Therefore, if you practice properly, you will eventually feel that your arms and palms are like a firm, solid, energetic mass. This creates a wonderful sensation of tingling warmth throughout your body, all the way to your fingertips.

The name of one of my 60 movements has been changed because sometimes the original names of Tai Chi Chuan movements were handed down by illiterate pugilists who did not speak the same dialect. Thus some of the names have been altered unintentionally. Movement number 21, called "pao hu kwai shan," may read: "Carrying the tiger back to the mountains." It seems to me that it has been misinterpreted and has lost its intended meaning. The original phrase reads: "Retreat to the mountain camp to prepare for a rematch." Since the old training camps were in the mountains, this phrase more accurately describes the actual movement. I feel that it is my duty as a Tai Chi Chuan practitioner to make this change and preserve the original meaning of these teachings, in spite of the criticism I may receive.

William C. C. Chen

I was born in Chekiang province, China, in 1935. Shortly after World War II, I moved to Taiwan with my family. As a teenager, I was very fascinated by all those imaginative martial arts novels, movies, and kung-fu handbooks popular with my generation. My most ambitious dream was to learn martial arts from a great master.

One day, my father took me to see his old-time playmate, Professor Cheng Man-ching, who was the best-known Tai Chi Chuan master. Very pleased to meet the son of his childhood friend, he asked if I would be interested in learning Tai Chi Chuan. I answered yes, with great delight.

A week later I became the youngest of Prof. Cheng's students. After a while I became deeply involved with Tai Chi Chuan. Besides relaxing my mind and body, it made me feel as if my inner energy were flowing throughout my entire body. My palms and fingertips were swollen with sensation, in harmony with my heartbeat. Such a wonderful feeling was beyond what any words could express. Soon, I fell deeply in love with this so-called "Supreme Ultimate Martial Art," and my progress sharply improved. Prof. Cheng was very proud of me and I became one of his favorite disciples.

For about a year I was assigned to the special internal training which is the most advanced part of training for Tai Chi Chuan. This was carried out three times a day—early morning, noon and late in the evening. Each day I arrived at his house early in the morning and did not leave until late at night. This full schedule gave me a great opportunity to understand his life style and martial arts skill. Every day I listened to his lectures and answers to questions about Tai Chi Chuan asked by students and visitors who streamed to his house. I realized the great advantage of staying in the master's house.

A few months after the special internal training, the brick fence of his house collapsed due to a combination of earthquake and typhoon. He asked if I would sleep over in a small training room at the back of his house to guard against the breaking-in of thieves. So I stayed in this small room—for almost three years.

This started my career in teaching Tai Chi Chuan. During the first year I stayed in his house, I was asked to teach beginners in their homes, thus getting pocket money as my remuneration. During the second year, in 1953, I was assigned to teach Tai Chi Chuan to the staff of the Postal and Telecommunications Administrative Agency of the government. A few months later I started another class in a branch of the Telecommunications Bureau. Soon after, I was also teaching at China Petroleum Company and Central Trust Bureau. This really kept me busy and earned me the title "Baby Master," since all those I taught were older than myself.

During those years I also took part in martial arts tournaments. In 1954 I was defeated. Two years later I was a member of the Taiwan group competing with experts from Hong Kong and Macao. Although I won at the beginning, I was eventually eliminated from the games. In 1958 I became fairly successful in the Chinese martial arts tournaments, becoming a winner in the light-weight division. I also gained recognition among Tai Chi Chuan enthusiasts in Singapore and Malaysia, so that in early 1959 I was invited to teach Tai Chi Chuan in Singapore, Malaysia, and later in Bangkok, Thailand.

In 1962 I enrolled as a student in the University of Hawaii right after I arrived at the paradise island of Oahu. There I was approached by various experts of Chinese martial arts for friendly matches, and in no time at all I began to give demonstrations. Within two weeks I was honored to teach as head instructor at the Honolulu Tai Chi Chuan Association. I also gave group and private classes in the community.

In 1963 I spent my entire summer vacation in San Francisco, where I gave a demonstration at the Chinatown Tai Chi Chuan Club. As a result I was asked to give instructions to the assistants there, and also to lecture to some of its masters. Dr. Lu Huiching, a noted instructor who was teaching a different style of this art at her Tai Chi Chuan studio on Teller Street in San Francisco, requested me to instruct her and her friends, and later her advanced students. She wrote a book called "A Manual of Instruction" on Tai Chi Chuan in 1974, giving me credit for my instruction.

Around the middle of 1965, Prof. Cheng Manching wrote me several times, asking me to teach at Springfield College in Springfield, Mass., and at the United Nations in New York City. After my arrival in New York, I turned down the Springfield offer because it was too far away. I also decided against teaching at the United Nations since it would mean depriving someone who was already there of his position. Instead, I opened a studio of my own, the William C. C. Chen School of Tai Chi Chuan, in the

Chelsea area of New York City. Later its name was changed to Tai Chi Chuan School, Inc.

For the public acceptance I have received in the United States I should thank many. Among them is Robert Smith, whose book, "Chinese Boxing," contains a chapter about me and my Tai Chi Chuan. Another is Master Aaron Banks, the greatest martial arts promoter in this country. He invited me to give exhibitions from his very first session of the Oriental World of Self-Defense in 1967 and for many subsequent years. I also thank Bronson Dudley, who, in an article in the August 1968 issue of *Black Belt,* called me "the Barnum of Brawl." As Tai Chi Chuan was quite new to Americans in the mid-1960's, all these things helped me gain acceptance not only in this country, but also in Europe and Australia.

Throughout all the years of my Tai Chi Chuan career, I have gained greatly in the knowledge and understanding of this unique form of martial art, which is one of the most effective for self-defense, as well as for physical fitness and mental well-being. I am really happy to share it with all those in my school and my workshops in different parts of the U.S.A. and Europe. I am happy that they appreciate my way of using the simplest, easiest and most common words, instead of the old terminology, to explain the mechanics and philosophy of Tai Chi Chuan.

Self Training

In the art of Tai Chi Chuan for self-defense, the best method to succeed is to practice a limited number of moves in slow motion each time. A beginner learning to type must practice slowly and properly. We must do so in Tai Chi Chuan as well as in so many other things in life.

The fewer the number of things that I try to learn, the more I am able to concentrate and the easier it becomes to perfect them. Practicing only a few movements at one time, combining slow motion with relaxation, were essential to the development of my learning process. This conditioned my mind and body slowly and correctly to have natural reflexes towards to the art of self defense.

After my daily practice of the Tai Chi Chuan forms, I broke down the form into a set of 4 or 5 movements to use as fighting techniques. I spent an additional hour to train in these techniques and repeated each of them 200 to 500 times in slow motion and with relaxation. This allowed me to focus my mind on the inner energy flow, coordinated with the outer action. Once I had repeated each technique 5000 times or more, the conditioning of these techniques reached a satisfactory level of performance in slow motion as well as at full speed. I then went on to the next set of movements, and so on.

Practicing in this manner, it took me nearly a year to complete Professor Cheng's short form of 37 postures. I worked on the movements again and again for many more years. Sometimes I chose a few movements and practiced them together as a combination technique, beginning with slow motion and speeding up afterwards. This again was done until the conditioning reached a satisfactory stage before moving on to the next set of combinations.

I was assigned to assist in Professor Cheng's internal training. This is training the body to absorb punches and kicks. During the second year, I followed the formula for training myself in my leisure time. After training an hour a day, in less than a year I found my body was able to take punches and kicks. This was of immense help to my free fighting training. Since I was able to train without fear of getting hurt, I could concentrate on good techniques as well as coordination. This added to my enjoyment in the art of self-defense.

Living in Professor Cheng's house was a priceless opportunity to obtain the right information for correct training. Even the few of us who were close disciples of Professor Cheng had little chance to see him practice the entire form of Tai Chi Chuan. However, we often saw him work on a few movements here and there. He never directly instructed me to train in this manner. But having gathered such valuable information this way, it appears to me that concentrating on a few movements at one time, and practicing in slow motion is the best way of conditioning to achieve the real art of Tai Chi Chuan.

There are many martial artists who have studied either soft styles or hard styles for a number of years without achieving real self-defense capability. Perhaps due to the impatient nature of man, they wanted to practice too many things and to have quick results.

By practicing a limited number of techniques, doing them in slow motion like the Tai Chi Chuan moves, repeating them until perfection, and then going on to the next technique. This would be the best method to reach the ultimate goal in the art of self-defense.

Definition of "Master"

In Tai Chi Chuan and other martial arts we often see the title of Master. How is this title conferred? Who is qualified to be called a master?

By implication, the term "master" indicates that a person has created a masterpiece and that his work is valued by a large number of people who know the particular subject. A masterpiece may be a work in art, music, literature or any other creative subject.

Naturally, every person feels and believes that his creations are good, great or even superb, but such a belief by itself does not qualify the person to be a master. They must also gain wide acceptance.

As in higher institutes of learning, one must complete a thesis to receive an academic degree. Simply by writing such a thesis one does not qualify for the degree he or she is seeking. It must be presented to the academic authorities for evaluation. For the same reason, an artist who has completed a painting, a composer who has written a symphony, or a writer who has written a book does not necessarily become a master. His work must also gain wide acceptance.

In China, there are many ways of addressing a teacher, whether of literature or martial arts. The following are the best known titles:

Sien-sun: " 先生 " Meaning "first born" or someone who was born before you, therefore who knows more than you.

Lao-sze: " 老師 " "Old teacher," which is used even on young people as "old" is a venerated term in China.

Chiao-sou: " 教授 " "Professor," usually used for

a teacher in a college or university.

Si-fu: " 師 父 " "Teacher-father." In traditional China, it has been the custom for a person's biological father to send his son to a teacher when the child was as young as five. This was usually done when the man wanted his son to learn some unusual skill from a famous teacher. The child would serve as an apprentice by living in the teacher's house, doing everything and behaving in every way as instructed by the teacher, who temporarily was also his father. Only when the child had learned the way of life as prescribed by his Si-fu, would the latter begin to teach him the skills. As a rule, such a teacher treated his students literally as disciples, always limiting the number from one to several. Today, such a practice is rare though still found here and there.

Si-fu: " 師 傅 " "Expert," means a qualified instructor or trainer, who has acquired special skills in or knowledge of a particular subject. It is an acceptable term for addressing a teacher in Chinese martial art circles and schools anywhere in the world. *Lao-sze* and *Sien-sun* are also acceptable terms in the Chinese community. The titles Doctor and Professor are used in the same sense as in the West. Of course, martial arts masters range widely in their degrees of educational background.

In the case of Professor Cheng Man-ching, since he taught Chinese painting in the College of Chinese Culture and Art in Shanghai, China, in his late twenties, he certainly has earned the title of "Professor." In my own case, it would be appropriate for my students to address me as Master, *Si-fu, Lao-sze* or *Sien-sun.*

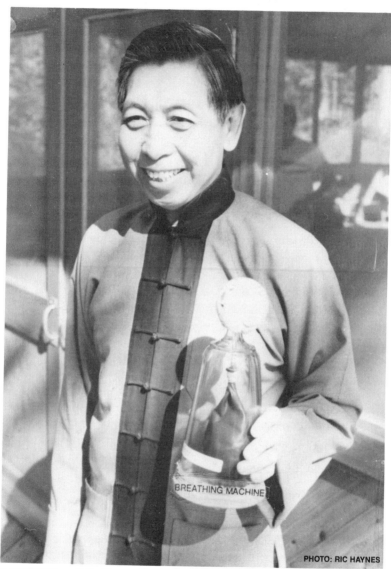

Author William C.C. Chen 陳王誠

KEY TO SYMBOLS

1. Illustration of the movements by photos:

   R = Weight on right leg.
   L = Weight on left leg.

   Broken line (_ _ _ _) represents the left side.
   Solid line (_____) represents the right side.

2. Description of the movements:

   The movements listed under a single number are normally performed simultaneously.

   For example: (as on page 46)

   2. Turn body 45° to the right.
      Move right foot one step to the back corner.
      Move right palm next to right hip, facing back.
      Move left palm 1½ feet away from left hip, facing up.

   Some of the movements under a single number are preceded by a dot (•). Perform all these movements simultaneously as a second action immediately after the undotted movement or movements.

   For example: (As on page 32)

   4. Shift weight to left leg 70%.
      • Turn body 20° to the left.
      • Move left palm next to left hip.
      • Move right palm forward to the front of right shoulder, facing out.

The Names of the Sixty Movements

1. Preparation
1 2 3

2. Beginning
1 2 3 4 5 6

3. Ward Off with Left Hand
1 2 3 4

4. Ward Off with Right Hand
1 2 3 4 5

5. Roll Away
1 2 3

6. Press
1 2

7. Push
1 2

8. Single Whip
1 2 3 4 5 6 7

9. Lifting the Hands
1 2 3

10. Shoulder Strike
1 2 3

11. White Crane Spreads
its Wing
1 2

12. Cross Over the Knee
and Step
1 2 3 4 5

13. Playing the Guitar
1 2 3

14. Cross Over the Knee
and Step
1 2 3 4

15. Step Up, Deflect,
Intercept and Punch
1 2 3 4 5 6

16. Get the Needle at the
Sea Bottom
1 2 3 4

17. Spread Arm like a Fan
1 2 3

18. Turn and Strike with
Back Fist, Chop with Fingers
1 2 3 4 5 6

19. Withdraw and Push
1 2 3 4 5

20. Crossing Hands
1 2 3 4 5 6

21. Retreat to Mountain Camp
for Rematch
1 2 3 4

22. Roll Away
1 2

23. Press
1 2

24. Push
1 2

25. Diagonal Single Whip
1 2 3 4 5 6 7

26. A Fist Under the Elbow
1 2 3 4 5

27. Step Back to Drive the
Monkey Away
1 2 3 4

28. Diagonal Flying Posture
1 2 3 4

29. Waving Hands in
the Clouds
1 2 3 4 5

30. Single Whip
1 2 3 4 5 6

3

31. Snake Creeps Down
    1 2 3 4

32. Golden Pheasant Stands on
    Left Leg
    1 2 3

33. Golden Pheasant Stands on
    Right Leg
    1 2

34. Kick with Right Foot
    1 2 3 4 5 6

35. Kick with Left Foot
    1 2 3 4 5

36. Turn Around and Strike
    with Heel
    1 2 3 4

37. Step Up and Strike
    with Fist
    1 2 3

38. Strike Ears with Fists
    1 2 3 4 5 6

39. Roll Away
    1 2

40. Press
    1 2

41. Push
    1 2

42. Single Whip
    1 2 3 4 5 6 7

43. Fair Lady at the Shuttle (1)
    1 2 3 4 5 6

44. Fair Lady at the Shuttle (2)
    1 2 3 4

45. Fair Lady at the Shuttle (3)
    1 2 3 4

46. Fair Lady at the Shuttle (4)
    1 2 3 4

47. Ward Off with Left Hand
    1 2 3 4

48. Ward Off with Right Hand
    1 2 3 4 5

49. Roll Away
    1 2 3

50. Press
    1 2

51. Push
    1 2

52. Single Whip
    1 2 3 4 5 6 7

53. Snake Creeps Down
    1 2 3 4

54. Step Up to Seven Stars
    of the Dipper
    1 2 3

55. Step Back to Ride the Tiger
    1 2 3

56. Turn Around with the Lotus
    Kick
    1 2 3 4 5

57. Bend the Bow to Shoot
    the Tiger
    1 2 3

58. Step Up, Deflect, Intercept
    and Punch
    1 2 3 4 5 6

59. Withdraw and Push
    1 2 3

60. Crossing Hands
    1 2 3 4 5 6

(1)
PREPARATION

1

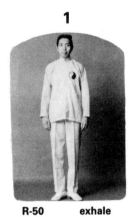

R-50   exhale

2   **3**

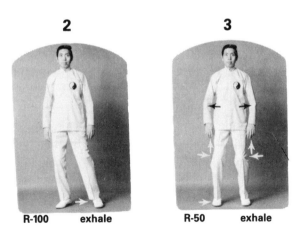

R-100   exhale   R-50   exhale

(1)
PREPARATION

1. Stand straight and relaxed, with heels together in a "V" position.

2. Shift weight to right leg 100%.
   - Move left foot one step to the left, toes pointing forward.

3. Shift weight to left leg 50%.
   - Turn right foot in slightly till the toes point forward, feet parallel.
   - Flex elbows slightly outward, with palms facing back.

(2)
BEGINNING

1

2

3

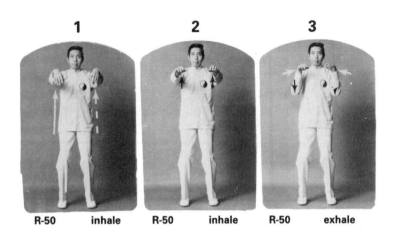

R-50 inhale	R-50 inhale	R-50 exhale

4

5

6

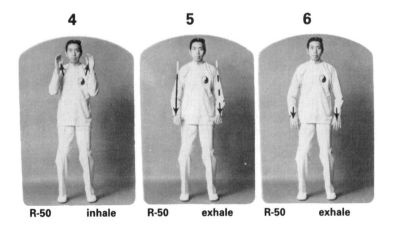

R-50 inhale	R-50 exhale	R-50 exhale

(2)
BEGINNING

1. Raise both wrists to shoulder level, arms extended, with hands hanging down.

2. Raise both palms to wrist level, facing down.

3. Draw both palms horizontally back toward the shoulder, as the elbows drop, palms still face down.

4. Raise both palms, until they face forward.

5. Drop both hands straight down next to the hips, palms facing down.

6. Drop both palms until they face back.

(3)
WARD OFF WITH LEFT HAND

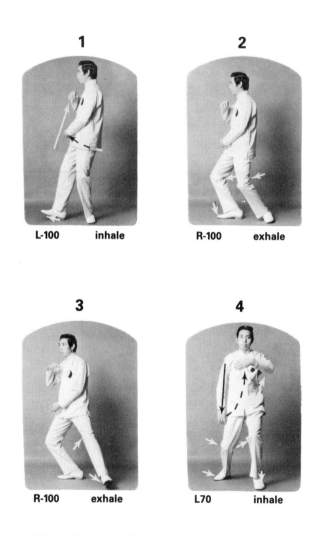

1

L-100   inhale

2

R-100   exhale

3

R-100   exhale

4

L70   inhale

(3)
WARD OFF WITH LEFT HAND

1. Shift weight to left leg 100%.

   Turn right foot out on the heel 90°.

   Turn body 90° to the right.

   Raise right palm in front of right chest, facing down.

   Move left palm in front of right hip joint, facing up. Both palms are facing each other.

2. Shift weight to right leg 100%, bending your knees slightly for the duration of the 60 postures.

3. Move left foot one step forward.

   Turn body 45° to the left.

4. Shift weight to left leg 70%.
   - Turn body another 45° to the left.
   - Raise left palm to the front of the solar plexus, facing in.
   - Drop right palm next to right hip, facing back.
   - Turn right foot in on the heel 45°.

(4)
WARD OFF WITH RIGHT HAND

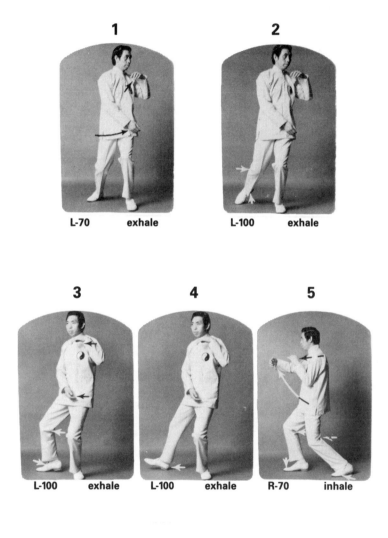

1

L-70 exhale

2

L-100 exhale

3

L-100 exhale

4

L-100 exhale

5

R-70 inhale

(4)
WARD OFF WITH RIGHT HAND

1. Turn body 25° to the left.
   Move left palm in front of left chest, facing down.
   Move right palm in front of left hip joint, facing up.
2. Shift weight to left leg 100%.
   Raise right heel, until only toes touch the ground.
3. Turn body 70° to the right.
   Turn right foot in on the toes 45°.
4. Move right foot one step forward.
5. Shift weight to right leg 70%.
   - Turn body 45° to the right.
   - Raise right palm to the front of the solar plexus, facing in.
   - Move left palm forward as the elbow drops, until the palm is between right palm and the body, facing forward.
   - Turn left foot in on the heel 45°.

(5)
ROLL AWAY

1

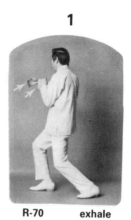

R-70   **exhale**

2

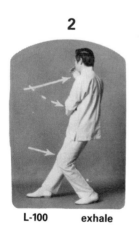

L-100   **exhale**

3

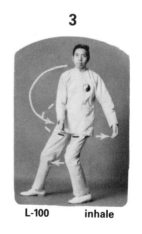

L-100   **inhale**

(5)
ROLL AWAY

1. Turn body and arms 25° to the right.
2. Shift weight back to left leg 100%.
   Draw right palm back, as the elbow drops, until the palm is in front of the shoulder, facing left.
   Move left palm in next to right elbow, facing up.
3. Turn body 115° to the left.
   Curve right palm down in front of left hip joint, facing back.
   Move left palm back, until the palm is 1½ feet behind the hip, facing forward.

(6)
PRESS

1

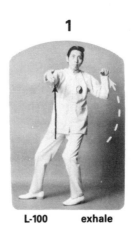

L-100   **exhale**

2

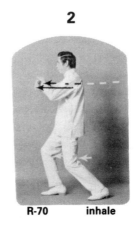

R-70   **inhale**

(6)
PRESS

1. Raise right palm to chest level, facing back.
   Curve left palm up to shoulder level, facing down.
2. Shift weight to right leg 70%.
   • Turn body 90° to the right.
   • Move right palm to the front of the solar plexus, facing in.
   • Move left palm forward to press right wrist lightly.

(7)
PUSH

1

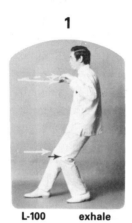

L-100   **exhale**

2

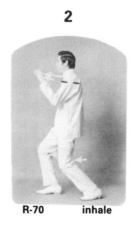

R-70   **inhale**

17

(7)
PUSH

1. Shift weight back to left leg 100%.
   Draw both palms back, as the elbows drop, until palms are right in front of the shoulder, facing down.

2. Shift weight to right leg 70%, then move forearms forward until palms are 1½ feet away from the shoulders, facing forward.

(8)
SINGLE WHIP

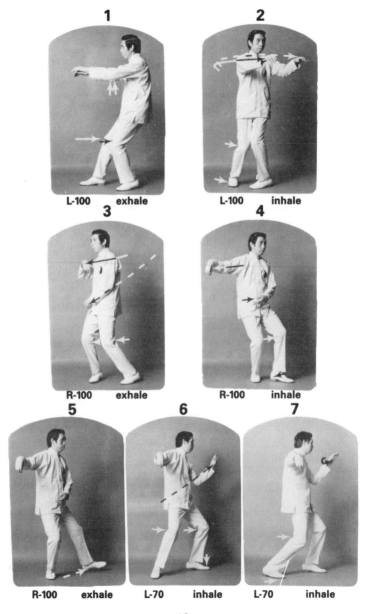

1

L-100   exhale

2

L-100   inhale

3

R-100   exhale

4

R-100   inhale

5

R-100   exhale

6

L-70   inhale

7

L-70   inhale

(8)
SINGLE WHIP

1. Shift weight back to left leg 100%.
   Move body back until arms are almost straight, palms are facing down.
2. Both arms follow as body turns 135° to the left.
   Turn right foot in on the heel 90°.
3. Shift weight to right leg 100%.
   Turn body 90° to the right.
   Move right hand in front of right chest, while drawing finger tips together and pointing them to the ground.
   Drop left palm in front of right hip joint, facing up.
4. Turn body 90° to the left.
   Turn left foot in on the ball of the foot 90°.
   Push right wrist out until the arm is almost straight.
5. Turn body 20° to the left.
   Move left foot one step to the left front.
6. Shift weight to left leg 70%.
   • Turn body 10° to the left.
   • Raise left palm to the front of left shoulder, facing in.
7. Turn left palm out, as body turns 15° to the left.
   Turn right foot in on the heel 45°.

LIFTING THE HAND

1

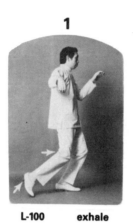

L-100   exhale

2

3

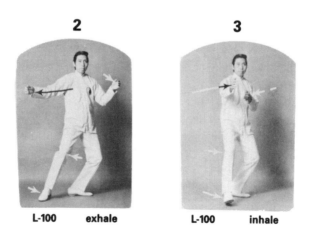

L-100   exhale   L-100   inhale

(9)
LIFTING THE HAND

1. Shift weight to left leg 100%.
   Raise right heel until the toes are lightly touching the ground.

2. Turn body 70° to the right.
   Turn left palm to face right.
   Open right hand into a palm as it turns to face left.
   Turn right foot in on the ball of the foot 90°.

3. Move right arm to the front of right shoulder.
   Move left palm to the front of the solar plexus, facing right elbow.
   Move right foot one step to the front of left heel, touching ground with right heel only.

(10)
SHOULDER STRIKE

1

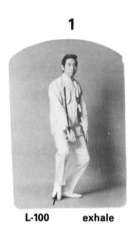

L-100   **exhale**

2

3

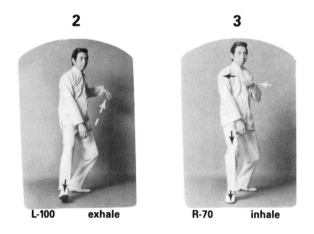

L-100   **exhale**   **R-70**   **inhale**

(10)
SHOULDER STRIKE

1. Turn body 45° to the left.
   Drop left palm next to left hip, facing right.
   Drop right palm in front of right hip joint, facing left.
   Move right foot one step back in front of left heel, touching ground with toes only.
2. Move right foot one step forward from left heel.
   Raise left palm to the back of left chest, facing down.
3. Shift weight to right leg 70%.
   Turn body 20° to the right.
   Move left palm in front of the solar plexus.
   Turn right elbow out to point slightly forward.

(11)
WHITE CRANE SPREADS ITS WING

1

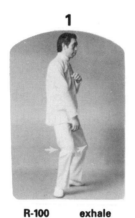

R-100   exhale

2

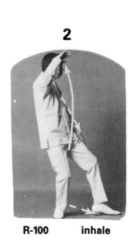

R-100   inhale

(11)
WHITE CRANE SPREADS ITS WING

1. Shift weight to right leg 100%.
   Turn body 50° to the left.
2. Move left foot one step to the front of right heel,
   touching ground with the ball of the foot only.
   Raise right palm next to right temple, facing out.
   Drop left palm next to left hip.

(12)
CROSS OVER THE KNEE AND STEP

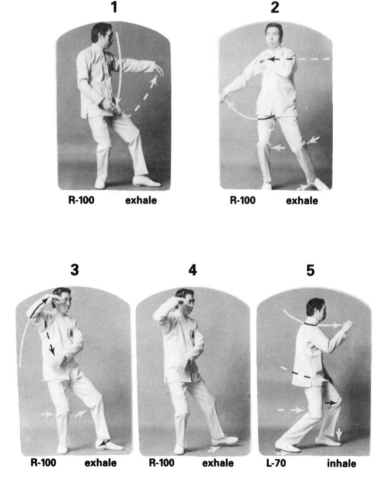

1

R-100   exhale

2

R-100   exhale

3

R-100   exhale

4

R-100   exhale

5

L-70   inhale

(12)
CROSS OVER THE KNEE AND STEP

1. Turn body 45° to the right.

   Drop right palm next to right hip, facing up.

   Raise left palm to the front of left shoulder, facing down.

2. Turn body 45° to the right.

   Move right palm back 1½ feet away from right hip, facing in.

   Move left palm in front of right chest.

3. Turn body 45° to the left.

   Raise right palm next to right temple, facing down.

   Drop left palm in front of right hip joint.

4. Turn body 25° to the left.

   Move left foot one step forward.

5. Shift weight to left leg 70%.
   - Turn body 20° to the left.
   - Move left palm next to left hip.
   - Move right palm forward to the front of right shoulder, facing out.
   - Turn right foot in on the heel 45°.

(13)
PLAYING THE GUITAR

1

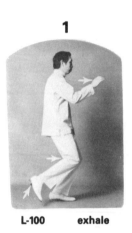

L-100   exhale

2

3

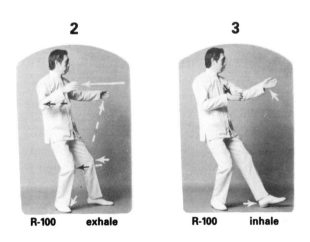

R-100   exhale   R-100   inhale

(13)
PLAYING THE GUITAR

1. Shift weight to left leg 100%.
   Raise right foot off the ground slightly.

2. Step down with right foot at the same spot as before and immediately shift weight to the right leg 100%.
   Raise left palm forward to chest level, facing right.
   Draw right palm in slightly as the elbow drops next to the ribs, facing left.

3. Turn body 20° to the right.
   Move left foot one step to the front of right heel, touching ground with left heel only.
   Move left arm to the front of the chest.
   Move right palm closer to left elbow.

(14)
CROSS OVER THE KNEE AND STEP

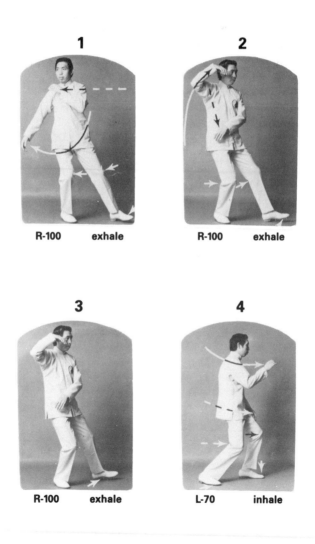

1

R-100   exhale

2

R-100   exhale

3

R-100   exhale

4

L-70   inhale

(14)
CROSS OVER THE KNEE AND STEP

1. Turn body 70° to the right.
   Drop right palm and move it back 1½ feet away from right hip, facing in.
   Move left palm in front of right chest, facing down.
2. Turn body 45° to the left.
   Raise right palm next to right temple, facing down.
   Drop left palm in front of right hip joint.
3. Turn body 25° to the left.
   Move left foot one step forward.
4. Shift weight to left leg 70%.
   • Turn body 20° to the left.
   • Move left palm next to left hip.
   • Move right palm forward to the front of right shoulder, facing out.

(15)
STEP UP, DEFLECT, INTERCEPT AND PUNCH

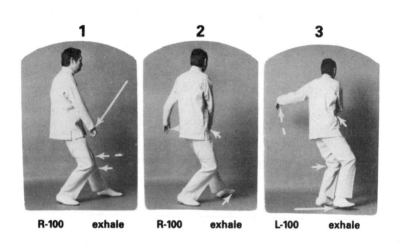

1	2	3
R-100 exhale	R-100 exhale	L-100 exhale

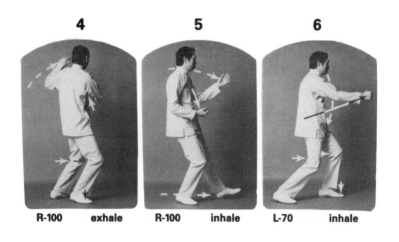

4	5	6
R-100 exhale	R-100 inhale	L-70 inhale

33

(15)
STEP UP, DEFLECT, INTERCEPT AND PUNCH

1. Shift weight back to right leg 100%.

   Change right palm into a fist as it drops in front of the groin, with knuckles facing forward.

2. Turn left foot out on the heel 45°, as body turns 30° to the left.

   Move left palm back 1 foot behind left hip, facing in.

3. Shift weight to left leg 100%, then move right foot forward a half-step from left arch at a 45° angle, as body turns 30° to the left.

   Move right fist back next to left waist.

   Move left palm back 1½ feet behind the waist.

4. Shift weight to right leg 100%.

   Raise right fist in front of left chest, with knuckle facing up.

   Raise left palm next to the face, facing out.

5. Move left foot one step forward, as body turns 90° to the right.

   Drop right fist to waist level, as the elbow drops, with knuckles facing down.

   Move left palm forward to the front of left shoulder, facing right.

6. Shift weight forward to left leg 70%.
   - Turn body 30° to the left.
   - Move left palm next to left hip, facing down.
   - Right fist punches forward to the front of the solar plexus, as a vertical fist.

(16)
GET THE NEEDLE AT SEA BOTTOM

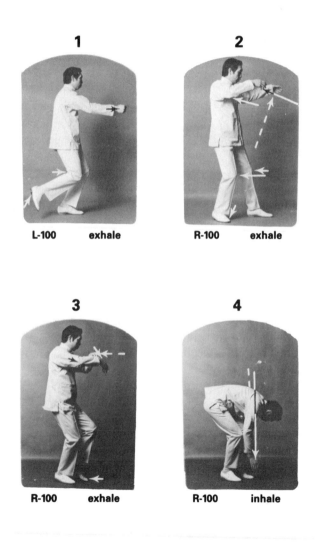

1

L-100   exhale

2

R-100   exhale

3

R-100   exhale

4

R-100   inhale

(16)
GET THE NEEDLE AT SEA BOTTOM

1. Shift weight to left leg 100%.
   Raise right foot off the ground slightly.

2. Step down with right foot at the same spot as before and immediately shift weight to right leg 100%.
   Raise left palm to the front of left shoulder, facing right.
   Raise right fist, changing it into a palm, to the front of the chest, fingers pointing to the ground.

3. Move left foot back in front of right heel, touching ground with the ball of the foot only.
   Move left palm inward until the fingers are lightly touching right wrist.

4. Bend body and arms down together until right finger tips are 5 inches from the ground.

(17)
SPREAD ARM LIKE A FAN

1

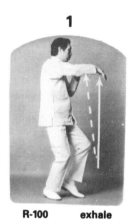

R-100   exhale

2   **3**

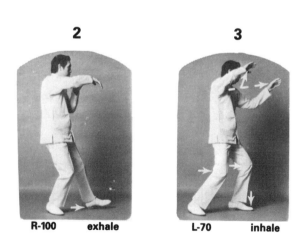

R-100   exhale   L-70   inhale

(17)
SPREAD ARM LIKE A FAN

1. Raise body and arms up, until the upper body is vertical.
2. Move left foot one step forward.
3. Shift weight to left leg 70%.
   Turn body 25° to the left.
   Move both hands to the front of left shoulder.
   • Turn body 50° to the right.
   • Move left fingers forward 1½ feet away from left shoulder, palm facing right.
   • Move right palm next to the right side of the face, facing out.

(18)
TURN AND STRIKE WITH BACK FIST

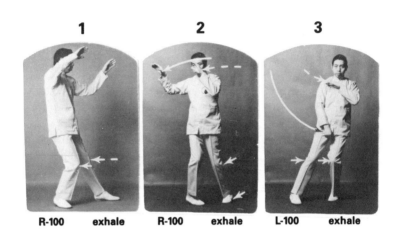

1	2	3
R-100 exhale	R-100 exhale	L-100 exhale

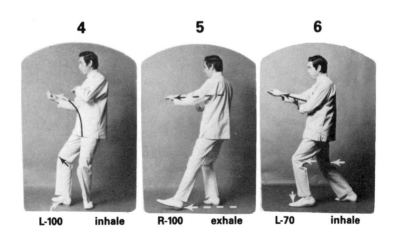

4	5	6
L-100 inhale	R-100 exhale	L-70 inhale

(18)
TURN AND STRIKE WITH BACK FIST

1. Shift weight back to right leg 100%.
2. Turn body 65° to the right.
   Turn left foot in on the heel 90°.
   Move left palm next to left temple, facing forward.
   Move right palm next to right temple, facing forward.
3. Shift weight to left leg 100%.
   Turn body 25° to the left.
   Move left palm in front of right chest, facing down.
   Change right palm into a fist, as it falls down to the front of right hip joint, with knuckles facing out.
4. Turn body ⁻70° to the right.
   Raise right foot off the ground and take a 180° twist step, touching the ground lightly.
   Swing right fist around as it follows the body turns to the right, until the fist is 1 foot away from the front of right chest, with knuckles facing down.
5. Shift weight to right leg 100%, then move left foot one step forward.
   Turn body 90° to the right.
   Move left palm forward 1½ feet away from left chest, facing down.
   Move right fist inward next to the waist, with knuckles facing down.
6. Shift weight to left leg 70%.
   • Turn body 45° to the left.
   • Move left palm inward to the front of right chest.
   • Open right fist into a palm as the fingers move forward 1½ feet away from chest, palm facing up.

(19)
WITHDRAW AND PUSH

1

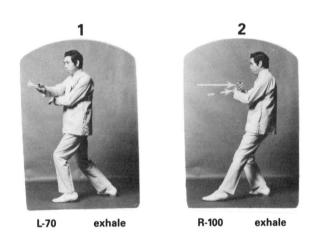

L-70   exhale   R-100   exhale

2

3   **4**   **5**

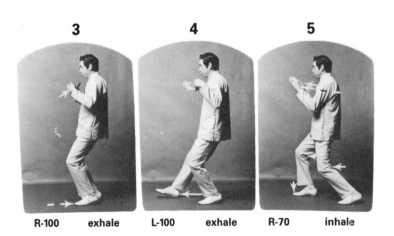

R-100   exhale   L-100   exhale   R-70   inhale

(19)
WITHDRAW AND PUSH

1. Turn body 30° to the left.
   Cross right arm over left wrist slightly.
2. Shift weight back to right leg 100%.
   Turn body 30° to the right.
   Draw right palm back, as the elbow drops, until both wrists are crossing each other, with palms facing in.
3. Move left foot back one step parallel to right foot at a 45° angle.
   Move palms back in front of the shoulders.
4. Shift weight to left leg 100%, then move right foot one step forward.
   Turn palms out.
5. Shift weight to right leg 70%.
   • Push palms forward 1½ feet away from the shoulders.

(20)
CROSSING HANDS

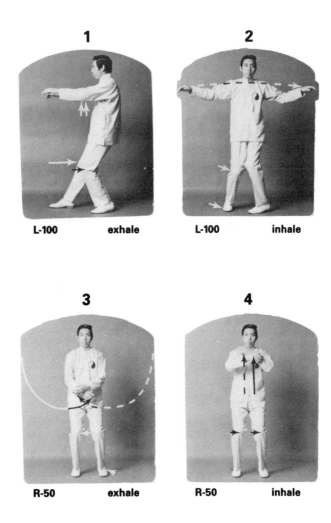

1

L-100   exhale

2

L-100   inhale

3

R-50   exhale

4

R-50   inhale

(20)
CROSSING HANDS

1. Shift weight back to left leg 100%.

   Move body back until arms are almost straight, palms are facing down.

2. Turn body 90° to the left.

   Move left arm across the front to the left side of the body.

   Turn right foot in on the heel 90°.

3. Shift weight to right leg 100%.
   - Move left foot back slightly until it is parallel to right foot, then shift weight back to left leg 50%.
   - Drop arms until right wrist crosses under left wrist in front of the stomach, palms are facing up.

4. Raise palms to the front of the chest, facing in.

(21)
RETREAT TO MOUNTAIN CAMP
FOR REMATCH

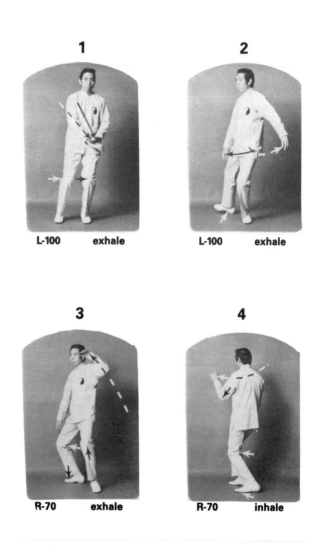

1

L-100   exhale

2

L-100   exhale

3

R-70   exhale

4

R-70   inhale

45

(21)
RETREAT TO MOUNTAIN CAMP
FOR REMATCH

1. Shift weight to left leg 100%.
   Drop palms together in front of left hip joint, while turning left palm up and turning right palm down.
2. Turn body 45° to the right.
   Move right foot one step to the back corner.
   Move right palm next to right hip, facing back.
   Move left palm 1½ feet away from left hip, facing in.
3. Shift weight to right leg 70%.
   Raise left palm next to the ear, facing down.
4. Turn body 90° to the right.
   Move left palm forward to the front of left shoulder, facing out.
   Turn right palm out.

(22)
ROLL AWAY

1

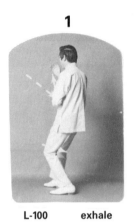

L-100   exhale

2

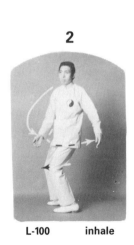

L-100   inhale

(22)
ROLL AWAY

1. Shift weight back to left leg 100%.
   Raise right palm in front of the shoulder, facing left.
   Move left palm in next to right elbow, facing up.
2. Turn body 90° to the left.
   Curve right palm down in front of left hip joint, facing back.
   Move left palm back, until the palm is 1½ feet behind the hip, facing forward.

(23)
PRESS

1

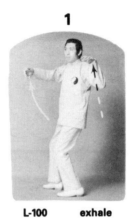

L-100   **exhale**

2

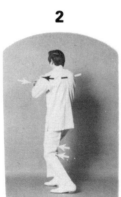

R-70   **inhale**

(23)
PRESS

1. Raise right palm to chest level, facing back.
   Curve left palm up to shoulder level, facing
   down.
2. Shift weight to right leg 70%.
   • Turn body 90° to the right.
   • Move right palm to the front of the solar plexus,
   facing in.
   • Move left palm forward to press right wrist
   lightly.

(24)
PUSH

1

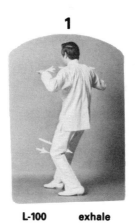

L-100   **exhale**

2

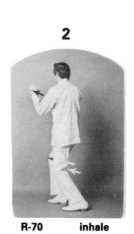

R-70   **inhale**

(24)
PUSH

1. Shift weight back to left leg 100%.

   Draw both palms back, as the elbows drop, until palms are right in front of the shoulder, facing down.

2. Shift weight to right leg 70%, then move forearms forward until palms are 1½ feet away from the shoulders, facing forward.

(25)
DIAGONAL SINGLE WHIP

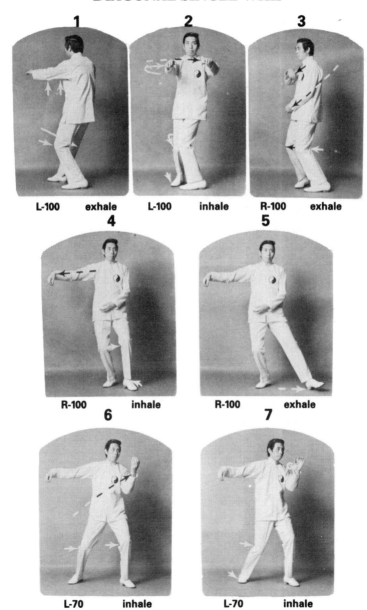

1 L-100 exhale
2 L-100 inhale
3 R-100 exhale
4 R-100 inhale
5 R-100 exhale
6 L-70 inhale
7 L-70 inhale

(25)
DIAGONAL SINGLE WHIP

1. Shift weight back to left leg 100%.
   Move body back until arms are almost straight, palms are facing down.
2. Both arms follow as body turns 135° to the left.
   Turn right foot in on the heel 90°.
3. Shift weight to right leg 100%.
   Turn body 90° to the right.
   Move right hand in front of right chest, while drawing finger tips together and pointing them to the ground.
   Drop left palm in front of right hip joint, facing up.
4. Turn body 90° to the left.
   Turn left foot in on the ball of the foot 90°.
   Push right wrist out until the arm is almost straight.
5. Turn body 20° to the left.
   Move left foot one step to the left corner.
6. Shift weight to left leg 70%.
   • Turn body 10° to the left.
   • Raise left palm to the front of left shoulder, facing in.
7. Turn left palm out, as body turns 15° to the left.
   Turn right foot in on the heel 45°.

(26)
A FIST UNDER THE ELBOW

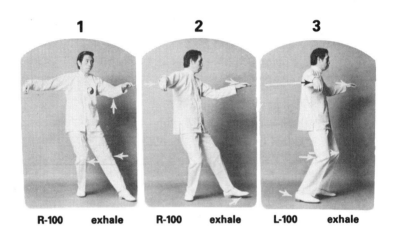

1	2	3
R-100 exhale	R-100 exhale	L-100 exhale

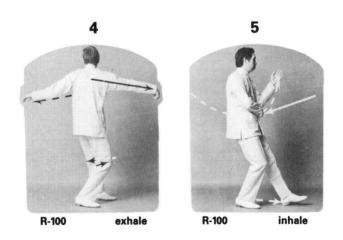

4	5
R-100 exhale	R-100 inhale

(26)
A FIST UNDER THE ELBOW

1. Shift weight back to right leg 100%.
   Move body back until left arm is almost straight, palm facing down.

2. Arms follow as body turns 25° to the left.
   Move left foot one step to the front of right heel.

3. Shift weight to left leg 100%.
   • Arms follow as body turns 20° to the left.
   • Move right foot one step to the right at 45° angle, the right arch is parallel to the left heel.

4. Shift weight to right leg 100%.
   Right arm follows as body turns 90° to the left.
   Move left arm to the back.

5. Turn body 90° to the right.
   Move left foot one step to the front of right heel, touching ground with left heel.
   Move left palm forward past the waist to the front of left shoulder, facing right.
   Change right hand into a fist as it moves beneath left elbow.

(27)
STEP BACK TO DRIVE THE MONKEY AWAY

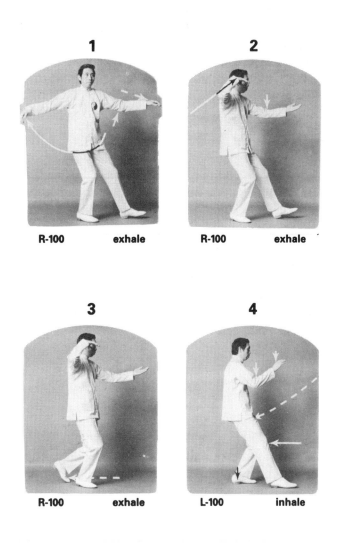

1

R-100 exhale

2

R-100 exhale

3

R-100 exhale

4

L-100 inhale

(27)
STEP BACK TO DRIVE THE MONKEY AWAY

1. Turn body 90° to the right.

   Extend left arm until it is almost straight, palm facing down.

   Change right fist into a palm, as it curves down to the back until it is 1½ feet away from right hip, facing in.

2. Turn body 45° to the left.

   Turn left palm face up.

   Curve right palm up next to right ear, facing down.

3. Turn body 20° to the left.

   Move left foot one step to the back, touching ground with toes only.

4. Shift weight to left leg 100%.
   - Turn body 25° to the left.
   - Drop left palm next to left hip, facing up.
   - Move right palm forward to the front of right shoulder, facing out.

(28)
DIAGONAL FLYING POSTURE

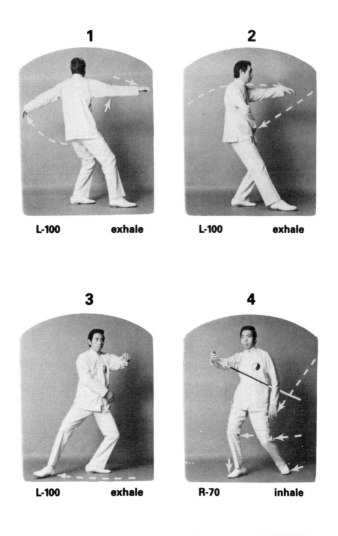

1

L-100   exhale

2

L-100   exhale

3

L-100   exhale

4

R-70   inhale

(28)
DIAGONAL FLYING POSTURE

1. Turn body 90° to the left.

   Curve left palm up to the back of left shoulder, facing down.

   Extend right palm until the arm is almost straight, facing down.

2. Turn body 90° to the right.

   Move left arm to the front of left shoulder.

   Drop right palm in front of left hip joint, facing in.

3. Left arm follows as body turns 45° to the right.

   Move right foot one step to the right corner.

4. Shift weight to right leg 70%.
   * Turn body 45° to the right
   * Drop left palm next to left hip.
   * Swing right arm up to the right corner until it is at shoulder level, palm facing up.

(29)
WAVING HANDS IN THE CLOUDS

1

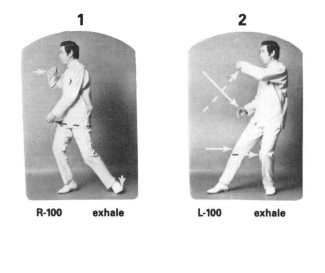

R-100   **exhale**

2

L-100   **exhale**

3

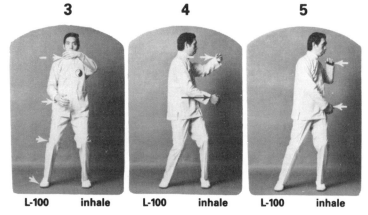

L-100   **inhale**

4

L-100   **inhale**

5

L-100   **inhale**

(29)
WAVING HANDS IN THE CLOUDS

1. Shift weight to right leg 100%.
   Turn body 45° to the right.
   Move left foot up slightly, until it is one foot apart parallel to right foot.
   Move left palm in front of right hip joint, facing up.
   Draw right palm in front of right chest, facing down.

2. Shift weight to left leg 100%.
   Raise left palm to neck level, facing in.
   Curve right palm out and down next to right hip, facing in.

3. Turn body 45° to the left.
   Turn right foot in on the heel 45°.
   Move palms to the front of the body.

4. Palms follow as body turns 45° to the left.

5. Draw left palm in front of left chest, facing down.
   Move right palm in front of left hip joint, facing up.

(30)
SINGLE WHIP

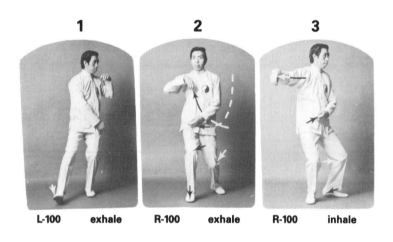

1	2	3
L-100 exhale	R-100 exhale	R-100 inhale

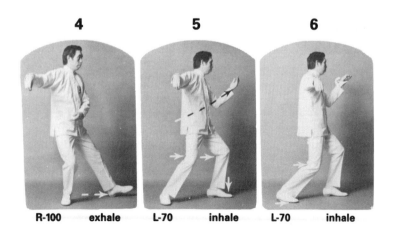

4	5	6
R-100 exhale	L-70 inhale	L-70 inhale

(30)
SINGLE WHIP

1. Move right foot one step forward.
2. Shift weight to right leg 100%.
   Turn body 90° to the right.
   Raise right hand in front of right chest, while drawing finger tips together and pointing them to the ground.
   Drop left palm in front of right hip joint, facing up.
3. Turn body 90° to the left.
   Turn left foot in on the ball of the foot 90°.
   Push right wrist out until the arm is almost straight.
4. Turn body 20° to the left.
   Move left foot one step to the left front.
5. Shift weight to left leg 70%.
   • Turn body 10° to the left.
   • Raise left palm to the front of left shoulder, facing in.
6. Turn left palm out, as body turns 15° to the left.
   Turn right foot in on the heel 45°.

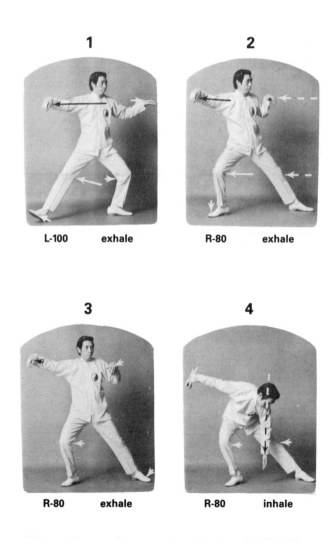

1

L-100   exhale

2

R-80   exhale

3

R-80   exhale

4

R-80   inhale

(31)
SNAKE CREEPS DOWN

1. Shift weight to left leg 100%.
   Turn body 45° to the right.
   Turn right foot out on the heel 90°.
   Extend left palm forward slightly, facing down.
2. Shift weight to right leg 80%.
   Draw left palm in front of left shoulder.
3. Turn body 45° to the right.
   Turn left foot in on the heel 45°.
   Fold left palm in until the fingers point to the ground.
4. Move left hand down, as the body bends, until the finger tips are 5 inches from the ground.

(32)
THE GOLDEN PHEASANT
STANDS ON LEFT LEG

1

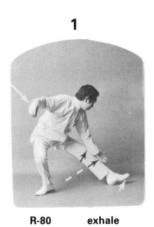

R-80   exhale

2

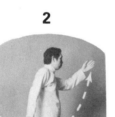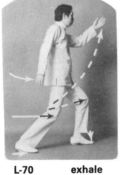

L-70   exhale

3

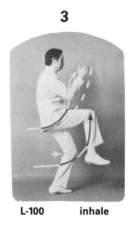

L-100   inhale

67

(32)
THE GOLDEN PHEASANT
STANDS ON LEFT LEG

1. Turn body 45° to the left.
   Turn left foot out on the heel 90°.
   Move left palm next to left shin, facing right.

2. Shift weight to left leg 70%.
   - Turn body 45° to the left.
   - Raise left palm to the face level.
   - Drop right grasped fingers right behind the hip.
   - Turn right foot in on the heel 90°.

3. Shift weight to left leg 100%.
   - Raise right knee to the hip level.
   - Change right hand into a palm, as it rises to the face level, facing left.
   - Drop left palm next to left hip, facing back.

(33)
THE GOLDEN PHEASANT
STANDS ON RIGHT LEG

1

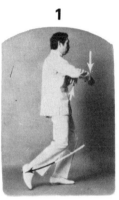

L-100   exhale

2

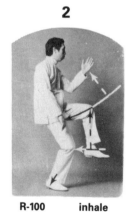

R-100   inhale

(33)
THE GOLDEN PHEASANT
STANDS ON RIGHT LEG

1. Step down with right foot one step to the back, touching ground with toes only.

   Raise left palm in front of the solar plexus, facing down.

   Drop right palm in front of left palm, facing down.

2. Shift weight to right leg 100%.
   • Raise left knee to the hip level.
   • Raise left palm to the face level, facing right.
   • Drop right palm next to right hip, facing back.

(34)
KICK WITH RIGHT FOOT

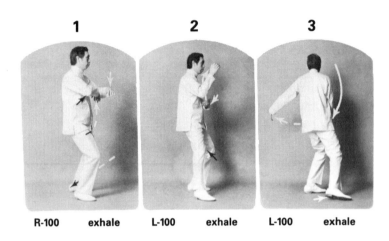

1   **2**   **3**

R-100   exhale   L-100   exhale   L-100   exhale

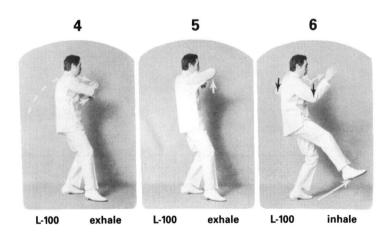

4   **5**   **6**

L-100   exhale   L-100   exhale   L-100   inhale

(34)
KICK WITH RIGHT FOOT

1. Step down with left foot one step to the left at 45° angle, touching ground lightly.

   Raise right palm in front of the solar plexus, facing down.

   Drop left palm in front of right palm, facing down.

2. Shift weight to left leg 100%.

   Raise right palm to the front of right shoulder, facing left corner.

   Move left palm next to right elbow, facing up.

3. Turn body 70° to the left.

   Move right foot one step to the right corner, touching ground with toes only.

   Move left palm back, until it is 1½ feet behind left hip, facing forward.

   Curve right palm down in front of left hip joint, facing back.

4. Turn body 25° to the right.

   Raise right palm to the front of left chest, facing in.

   Raise left wrist from the back and curve it down to the front, until it touches top of right wrist, palm facing in.

5. Raise both elbows slightly as the palms turn out, until right wrist is on top of left wrist.

6. Move right palm out as the elbow drops, until it is 1½ feet away from the face, facing left corner.

   Move left palm out as the elbow drops, until it is behind left ear, facing left corner.

   Kick right foot up towards right corner, until it is at knee level.

KICK WITH LEFT FOOT

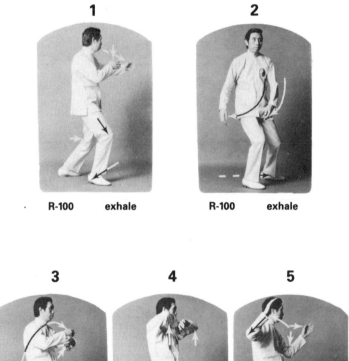

1

R-100   exhale

2

R-100   exhale

3

R-100   exhale

4

R-100   exhale

5

R-100   inhale

(35)
KICK WITH LEFT FOOT

1. Step down with right foot one step to right corner
   and immediately shift weight to· the right leg
   100%.

   Extend left palm out and down to the shoulder
   level, facing right corner.

   Drop right palm to the front of the solar plexus,
   facing left elbow.

2. Turn body 115° to the right.

   Move left foot one step to the left corner, touching
   ground with toes only.

   Move right palm back, until it is 1½ fｃet behind
   right hip, facing forward.

   Curve left palm down in front of right hip joint,
   facing back.

3. Turn body 25° to the left.

   Raise left palm to the front of right chest, facing
   in.

   Raise right wrist from the back and curves down
   to the front, until it touches top of left wrist, palm
   facing in.

4. Raise both elbows slightly as the palms turn out,
   until left wrist is on top of right wrist.

5. Move left palm out as the elbow drops, until it is
   1½ feet away from the face, facing right corner.

   Move right palm out as the elbow drops, until it is
   behind right ear, facing right corner.

   Kick left foot up towards left corner, until it is at
   knee level.

TURN AROUND AND STRIKE WITH HEEL

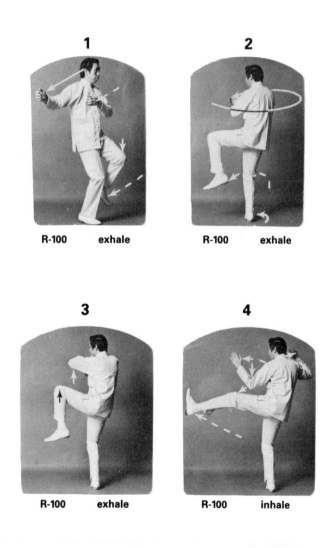

1

R-100   exhale

2

R-100   exhale

3

R-100   exhale

4

R-100   inhale

TURN AROUND AND STRIKE WITH HEEL

1. Turn body 45° to the right.

   Move left palm in front of right chest, facing in.

   Drop right palm to the chest level as the arm swings to the back, facing right corner.

   Swing left knee 135° to the right, as the leg folds in, but the foot still is off the ground.

2. Swing body around 225° counter-clockwise on the heel, as right foot turns around 135° and swing left knee around 270°.

   Right palm follows as the body swings around, until right wrist crosses over the top of left wrist.

3. Raise both elbows slightly as the palms turn out, until left wrist is on top of right wrist.

   Raise left knee to the front of the stomach.

4. Move left palm forward to the front of the face, as the elbow drops, facing right.

   Move right palm out as the elbow drops, until it is behind right ear, facing right corner.

   Kick left heel forward to the stomach level, until the leg is almost straight.

STEP UP AND STRIKE WITH FIST

1

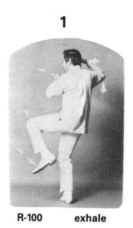

R-100   exhale

2   **3**

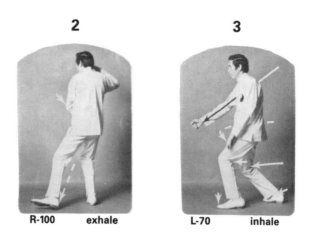

R-100   exhale   L-70   inhale

(37)
STEP UP AND STRIKE WITH FIST

1. Drop left foot next to right knee.

   Move left palm in front of right chest, facing down.

   Move right palm next to right temple, facing down.

2. Step down with left foot one step forward.

   Drop left palm down in front of right hip joint.

3. Shift weight forward to left leg 70%.
   - Turn body 45° to the left.
   - Move left palm next to left hip.
   - Change right palm into a vertical fist, as it punches forward at groin level.

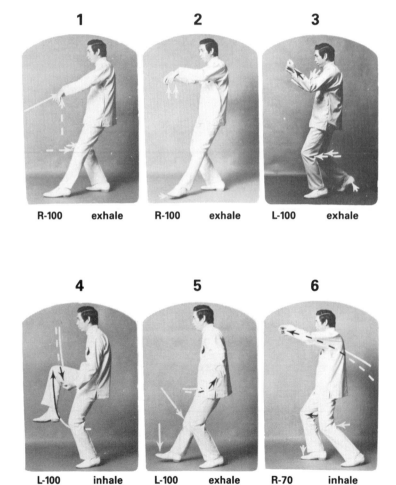

1	2	3
R-100 exhale	R-100 exhale	L-100 exhale

4	5	6
L-100 inhale	L-100 exhale	R-70 inhale

(38)
STRIKE EARS WITH FISTS

1. Shift weight back to right leg 100%.
   Change right fist into a palm as it moves to the front of the waist, facing down.
   Move left palm to the front of the waist, facing down.

2. Turn left foot out on the heel 45°.
   Raise both palms evenly to the chest level.

3. Shift weight forward to left leg 100%.
   Raise right heel until only toes touch the ground.
   Change both palms into fists, as they rise to face level, with both knuckles facing down.

4. Kick right knee up to the stomach level.
   Drop both fists next to the hips.

5. Step down with right foot one step forward.
   Move both fists out to the side of the body, until fists are 2 feet away from the waist, with both knuckles facing out.

6. Shift weight forward to right leg 70%, then the fists curve forward to strike opponent's ears, with both knuckles facing up.

(39)
ROLL AWAY

1

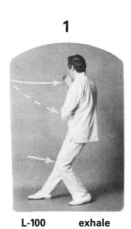

L-100   **exhale**

2

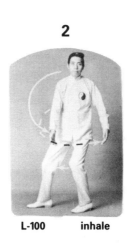

L-100   **inhale**

(39)
ROLL AWAY

1. Shift weight back to left leg 100%.

   Change right fist into a palm as the elbow drops, until the palm is in front of the shoulder, facing left.

   Change left fist into a palm as it drops in next to right elbow, facing up.

2. Turn body 90° to the left.

   Curve right palm down in front of left hip joint, facing back.

   Move left palm back, until the palm is 1½ feet behind the hip, facing forward.

(40)
PRESS

1

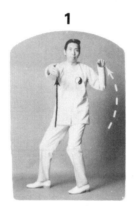

L-100   **exhale**

2

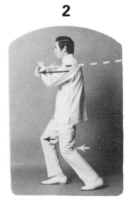

R-70   **inhale**

(40)
PRESS

1. Raise right palm to chest level, facing back.
   Curve left palm up to shoulder level, facing down.

2. Shift weight to right leg 70%.
   • Turn body 90° to the right.
   • Move right palm to the front of the solar plexus, facing in.
   • Move left palm forward to press right wrist lightly.

(41)
PUSH

1

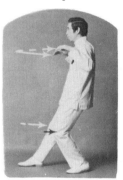

L-100   **exhale**

2

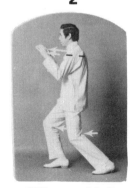

R-70   **inhale**

(41)
PUSH

1. Shift weight back to left leg 100%.
   Draw both palms back, as the elbows drop, until palms are right in front of the shoulder, facing down.
2. Shift weight to right leg 70%, then move forearms forward until palms are 1½ feet away from the shoulders, facing forward.

(42)
SINGLE WHIP

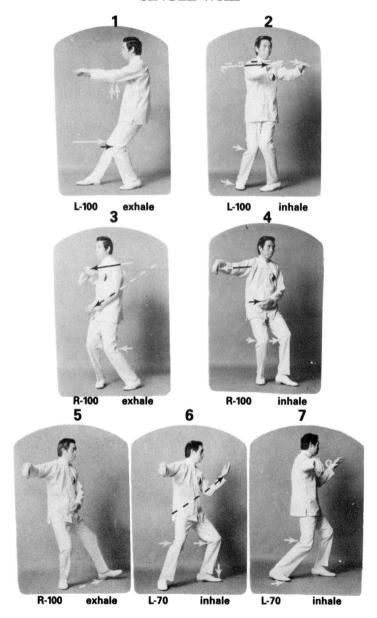

1 — L-100   exhale

2 — L-100   inhale

3 — R-100   exhale

4 — R-100   inhale

5 — R-100   exhale

6 — L-70   inhale

7 — L-70   inhale

(42)
SINGLE WHIP

1. Shift weight back to left leg 100%.
   Move body back until arms are almost straight, palms are facing down.

2. Both arms follow as body turns 135° to the left.
   Turn right foot in on the heel 90°.

3. Shift weight to right leg 100%.
   Turn body 90° to the right.
   Move right hand in front of right chest, while drawing finger tips together and pointing them to the ground.
   Drop left palm in front of right hip joint, facing up.

4. Turn body 90° to the left.
   Turn left foot in on the ball of the foot 90°.
   Push right wrist out until the arm is almost straight.

5. Turn body 20° to the left.
   Move left foot one step to the left front.

6. Shift weight to left leg 70%.
   • Turn body 10° to the left.
   • Raise left palm to the front of left shoulder, facing in.

7. Turn left palm out, as body turns 15° to the left.
   Turn right foot in on the heel 45°.

(43)
FAIR LADY AT THE SHUTTLE

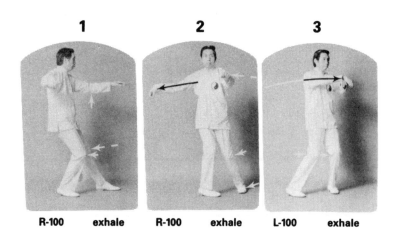

1	2	3
R-100 exhale	R-100 exhale	L-100 exhale

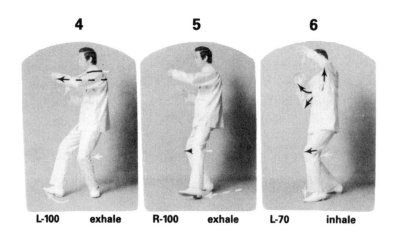

4	5	6
L-100 exhale	R-100 exhale	L-70 inhale

89

(43)
FAIR LADY AT THE SHUTTLE

1. Shift weight back to right leg 100%.
   Move body back until left arm is almost straight, facing down.

2. Both arms follow as body turns 90° to the right.
   Turn left foot in on the heel 90°.

3. Shift weight to left leg 100%.
   Turn body 45° to the left.
   Move right forearm to cross over left forearm.

4. Turn body 90° to the right.
   Turn right foot out on the heel 180°.
   Change right hand into a palm and move it in front of the solar plexus as the palm turns up.
   Turn left palm in.

5. Shift weight to right leg 100%.
   • Turn body 45° to the right.
   • Move left foot one step to the left corner.

6. Shift weight to left leg 70%.
   • Turn body 45° to the left.
   • Raise left palm in front of the forehead, as the palm turns out.
   • Move right palm forward, as it turns out.
   • Turn right foot in on the heel 45°.

(44)
FAIR LADY AT THE SHUTTLE (2)

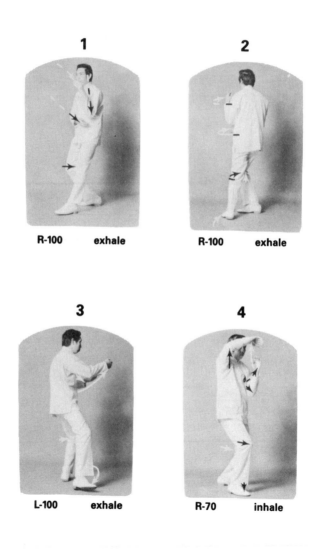

1

R-100   exhale

2

R-100   exhale

3

L-100   exhale

4

R-70   inhale

(44)
FAIR LADY AT THE SHUTTLE (2)

1. Shift weight back to right leg 100%.
   Move left palm to the front of left shoulder as elbow drops, facing right corner.
   Drop right palm next to left elbow, facing up.
2. Turn body 135° to the right.
   Turn left foot in on the heel 120°.
3. Shift weight to left leg 100%.
   • Turn body 45° to the right.
   • Move right foot one step to the back corner.
   • Drop left palm in front of the solar plexus, facing up.
   • Raise right palm to the front of left shoulder, facing in.
4. Shift weight to right leg 70%.
   • Turn body 90° to the right.
   • Raise right palm in front of the forehead, as the palm turns out.
   • Move left palm forward, as it turns out.
   • Turn left foot in on the heel 105°.

(45)
FAIR LADY AT THE SHUTTLE (3)

1

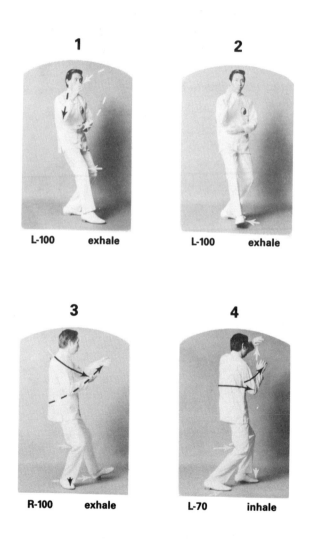

L-100   exhale

2

L-100   exhale

3

R-100   exhale

4

L-70   inhale

(45)
FAIR LADY AT THE SHUTTLE (3)

1. Shift weight back to left leg 100%.
   Move right palm to the front of right shoulder as elbow drops, facing left corner.
   Drop left palm next to right elbow, facing up.

2. Turn body 45° to the right.
   Turn right foot out on the heel 45°.

3. Shift weight to right leg 100%.
   - Turn body 45° to the left.
   - Move left foot one step to the left corner.
   - Drop right palm in front of the solar plexus, facing up.
   - Raise left palm to the front of right shoulder, facing in.

4. Shift weight to left leg 70%.
   - Turn body 90° to the left.
   - Raise left palm in front of the forehead, as the palm turns out.
   - Move right palm forward, as it turns out.
   - Turn right foot in on the heel 90°.

(46)
FAIR LADY AT THE SHUTTLE (4)

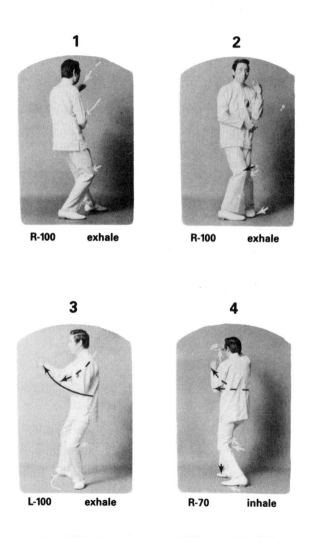

1

R-100   exhale

2

R-100   exhale

3

L-100   exhale

4

R-70   inhale

(46)
FAIR LADY AT THE SHUTTLE (4)

1. Shift weight back to right leg 100%.
   Move left palm to the front of left shoulder as elbow drops, facing right corner.
   Drop right palm next to left elbow, facing up.

2. Turn body 135° to the right.
   Turn left foot in on the heel 120°.

3. Shift weight to left leg 100%.
   • Turn body 45° to the right.
   • Move right foot one step to the back corner.
   • Drop left palm in front of the solar plexus, facing up.
   • Raise right palm to the front of left shoulder, facing in.

4. Shift weight to right leg 70%.
   • Turn body 90° to the right.
   • Raise right palm in front of the forehead, as the palm turns out.
   • Move left palm forward, as it turns out.
   • Turn left foot in on the heel 105°.

(47)
WARD OFF WITH LEFT HAND

1

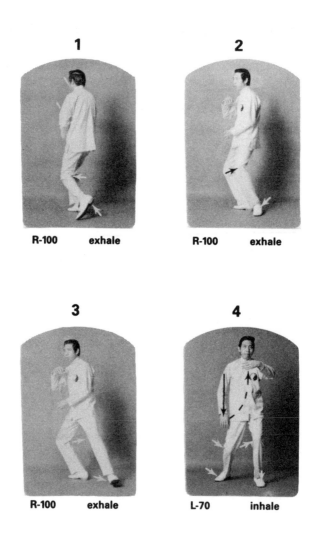

R-100   exhale

2

R-100   exhale

3

R-100   exhale

4

L-70   inhale

(47)
WARD OFF WITH LEFT HAND

1. Shift weight to right leg 100%.
   Drop right palm in front of right chest, facing down.
   Drop left palm in front of right hip joint, facing up. Both palms are facing each other.
   Raise left heel until the toes are lightly touching the ground.

2. Turn body 45° to the left.
   Turn left foot in on the toes 90°.

3. Move left foot one step forward.
   Turn body 45° to the left.

4. Shift weight to left leg 70%.
   • Turn body another 45° to the left.
   • Raise left palm to the front of the solar plexus, facing in.
   • Drop right palm next to right hip, facing back.
   • Turn right foot in on the heel 90°.

(48)
WARD OFF WITH RIGHT HAND

1

2

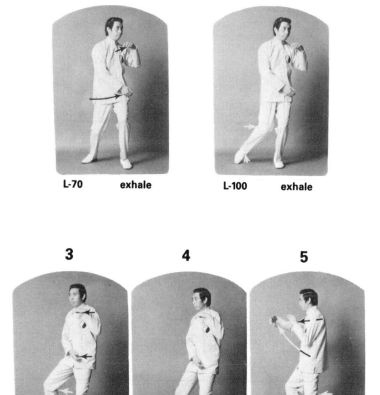

L-70   exhale

L-100   exhale

3

4

5

L-100   exhale

L-100   exhale

R-70   inhale

(48)
WARD OFF WITH RIGHT HAND

1. Turn body 25° to the left.
   Move left palm in front of left chest, facing down.
   Move right palm in front of left hip joint, facing up.
2. Shift weight to left leg 100%.
   Raise right heel, until only toes touch the ground.
3. Turn body 70° to the right.
   Turn right foot in on the toes 45°.
4. Move right foot one step forward.
5. Shift weight to right leg 70%.
   • Turn body 45° to the right.
   • Raise right palm to the front of the solar plexus, facing in.
   • Move left palm forward as the elbow drops, until the palm is between right palm and the body, facing forward.
   • Turn left foot in on the heel 45°.

(49)
ROLL AWAY

1

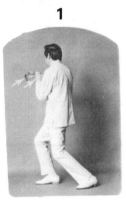

R-70   exhale

2   **3**

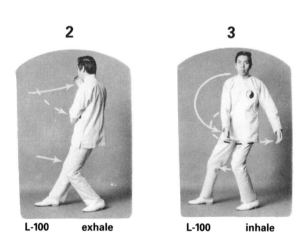

L-100   exhale   L-100   inhale

(49)
ROLL AWAY

1. Turn body and arms 25° to the right.
2. Shift weight back to left leg 100%.
   Draw right palm back, as the elbow drops, until the palm is in front of the shoulder, facing left.
   Move left palm in next to right elbow, facing up.
3. Turn body 115° to the left.
   Curve right palm down in front of left hip joint, facing back.
   Move left palm back, until the palm is 1½ feet behind the hip, facing forward.

(50)
PRESS

1

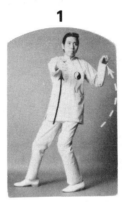

L-100   **exhale**

2

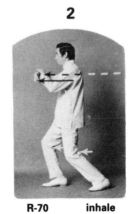

R-70   **inhale**

(50)
PRESS

1. Raise right palm to chest level, facing back.
   Curve left palm up to shoulder level, facing down.

2. Shift weight to right leg 70%.
   - Turn body 90° to the right.
   - Move right palm to the front of the solar plexus, facing in.
   - Move left palm forward to press right wrist lightly.

(51)
PUSH

1

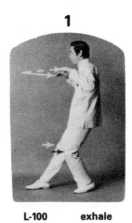

L-100   **exhale**

2

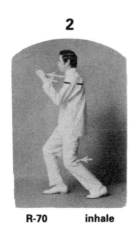

R-70   **inhale**

(51)
PUSH

1. Shift weight back to left leg 100%.
   Draw both palms back, as the elbows drop, until palms are right in front of the shoulder, facing down.
2. Shift weight to right leg 70%, then move forearms forward until palms are 1½ feet away from the shoulders, facing forward.

(52)
SINGLE WHIP

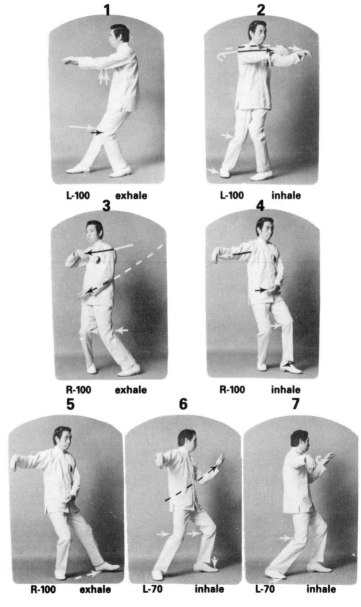

1

L-100   exhale

2

L-100   inhale

3

R-100   exhale

4

R-100   inhale

5

R-100   exhale

6

L-70   inhale

7

L-70   inhale

(52)
SINGLE WHIP

1. Shift weight back to left leg 100%.
   Move body back until arms are almost straight, palms are facing down.

2. Both arms follow as body turns 135° to the left.
   Turn right foot in on the heel 90°.

3. Shift weight to right leg 100%.
   Turn body 90° to the right.
   Move right hand in front of right chest, while drawing finger tips together and pointing them to the ground.
   Drop left palm in front of right hip joint, facing up.

4. Turn body 90° to the left.
   Turn left foot in on the ball of the foot 90°.
   Push right wrist out until the arm is almost straight.

5. Turn body 20° to the left.
   Move left foot one step to the left front.

6. Shift weight to left leg 70%.
   • Turn body 10° to the left.
   • Raise left palm to the front of left shoulder, facing in.

7. Turn left palm out, as body turns 15° to the left.
   Turn right foot in on the heel 45°.

(53)
SNAKE CREEPS DOWN

1

2

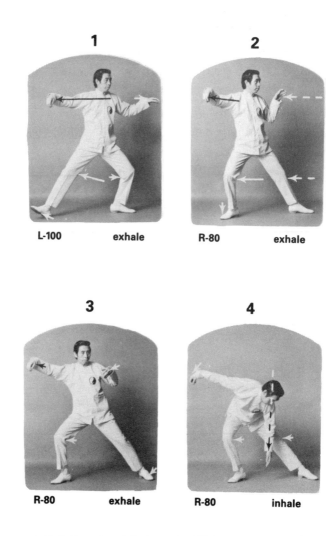

L-100   exhale

R-80   exhale

3

4

R-80   exhale

R-80   inhale

(53)
SNAKE CREEPS DOWN

1. Shift weight to left leg 100%.
   Turn body 45° to the right.
   Turn right foot out on the heel 90°.
   Extend left palm forward slightly, facing down.
2. Shift weight to right leg 80%.
   Draw left palm in front of left shoulder.
3. Turn body 45° to the right.
   Turn left foot in on the heel 45°.
   Fold left palm in until the fingers point to the ground.
4. Move left hand down, as the body bends, until the finger tips are 5 inches from the ground.

STEP UP TO SEVEN STARS OF THE DIPPER

1

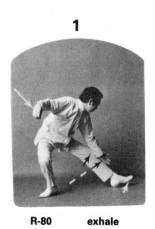

R-80   exhale

2   **3**

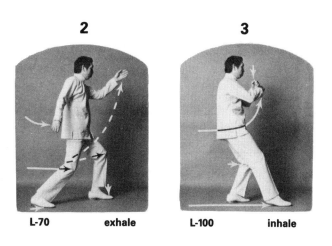

L-70   exhale   L-100   inhale

(54)
STEP UP TO SEVEN STARS OF THE DIPPER

1. Turn body 45° to the left.
   Turn left foot out on the heel 90°.
   Move left palm next to left shin, facing right.
2. Shift weight to left leg 70%.
   - Turn body 45° to the left.
   - Raise left palm to the face level.
   - Drop right grasped fingers right behind the hip.
   - Turn right foot on the heel 90°.
3. Shift weight to left leg 100%.
   - Move right foot one step forward, touching ground with the ball of the foot only.
   - Change left palm into a fist, as the wrist moves to the front of the chest.
   - Change right hand into a fist, as the wrist rises right in front of left wrist, both wrists are touching lightly.

(55)
STEP BACK TO RIDE THE TIGER

1

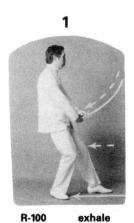

R-100   exhale

2

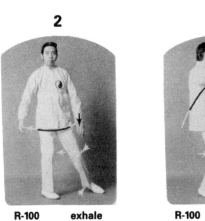

R-100   exhale

3

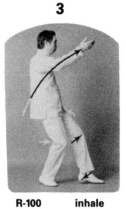

R-100   inhale

113

(55)
STEP BACK TO RIDE THE TIGER

1. Move right foot one step to the back at a 45° angle and immediately shift weight to the right leg 100%.

   Change both fists into palms, turn right palm up and left palm down, as they drop in front of the stomach, both wrists are still touching together.

2. Turn body 60° to the right.

   Raise left heel until only the toes touch the ground as the heel turns out 80°.

   Move right palm back 1½ feet behind right hip, facing in.

   Move left palm next to left hip, facing back.

3. Turn body 60° to the left.

   Swing right palm up to the front of the face, facing up.

   Move left foot one step to the front of right heel, touching ground with the ball of the foot only.

(56)
TURN AROUND WITH LOTUS KICK

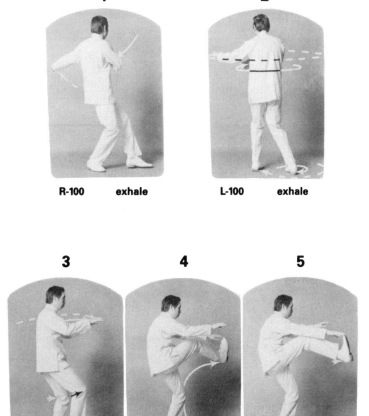

1

R-100   exhale

2

L-100   exhale

3

L-100   exhale

4

L-100   inhale

5

L-100   inhale

(56)
TURN AROUND WITH LOTUS KICK

1. Turn body 30° to the left.

   Move left palm out to the left rear corner until to the chest level, facing forward.

   Move right palm in front of left chest, facing in.

2. Swing body around 300° clockwise, as right foot turns in on the ball of right foot 225°, and swing around both arms 360° as the body turns.

   Sweep left foot around from front to the back at a 45° angle behind right toes, and immediately shift weight to left leg 100%.

3. Turn body 90° to the right, as right foot turns in on the ball of the foot 90°.

   Move both palms to the front of the shoulders, facing down.

4. Raise right foot to touch left palm.

5. Move right foot rightward to touch right palm.

(57)
BEND THE BOW TO SHOOT THE TIGER

1

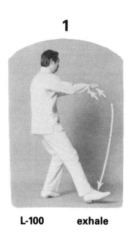

L-100   exhale

2

3

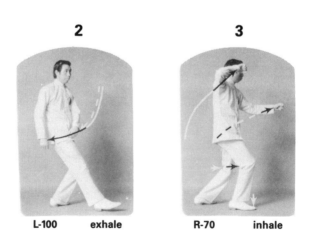

L-100   exhale   R-70   inhale

(57)
BEND THE BOW TO SHOOT THE TIGER

1. Step down with right foot one step forward.
   Turn body 25° to the left.
   Move both palms leftward slightly.
2. Turn body 70° to the right.
   Change right palm into a fist, as it drops back one foot behind right hip.
   Change left palm into a fist, as it drops in front of right hip joint.
3. Shift weight to right leg 70%.
   • Turn body 45° to the left.
   • Swing right fist up to the front of right temple.
   • Move left fist out to the front of left waist.

(58)
STEP UP, DEFLECT, INTERCEPT AND PUNCH

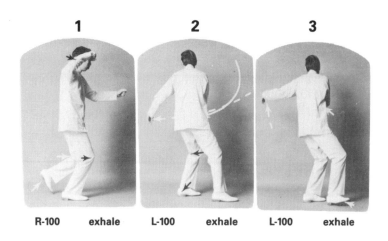

1 R-100   exhale
2 L-100   exhale
3 L-100   exhale

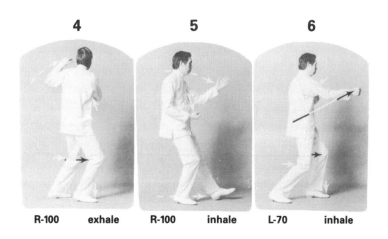

4 R-100   exhale
5 R-100   inhale
6 L-70   inhale

STEP UP, DEFLECT, INTERCEPT AND PUNCH

1. Shift weight to right leg 100%.
   Raise left foot off the ground slightly.

2. Step down with left foot at same spot as before, and immediately shift weight to left leg 100%, as body turns 60° to the left.
   Drop right fist in front of the groin, with kunckle facing out.
   Change left fist into a palm, as it moves back one foot behind left hip, facing in.

3. Move right foot half step back towards left arch at a 45° angle.
   Move right fist next to left waist.
   Move left palm back 1½ feet behind the waist.

4. Shift weight to right leg 100%.
   Raise right fist in front of left chest, with knuckle facing up.
   Raise left palm next to the face, facing out.

5. Move left foot one step forward, as body turns 90° to the right.
   Drop right fist to waist level, as the elbow drops, with knuckles facing down.
   Move left palm to the front of left shoulder, facing right.

6. Shift weight forward to left leg 70%.
   • Turn body 30° to the left as it moves forward, until left palm is in front of the chest.
   • Right fist punches forward to the front of the solar plexus, as a vertical fist.

(59)
WITHDRAW AND PUSH

1

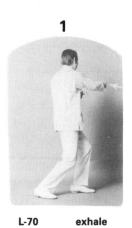

L-70   exhale

2

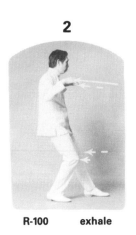

R-100   exhale

3

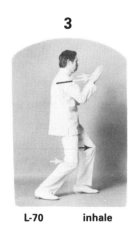

L-70   inhale

(59)
WITHDRAW AND PUSH

1. Turn body 30° to the left.
   Move left palm down slightly, as right elbow crosses it over.

2. Shift weight back to right leg 100%.
   Turn body 30° to the right.
   Change right fist into a palm as it draws in front of right shoulder, facing down.
   Draw left palm in front of left shoulder, facing down.

3. Shift weight to left 70%, then move forearms forward until palms are 1½ feet away from the shoulders, palms are facing forward.

(60)
CROSSING HANDS

1

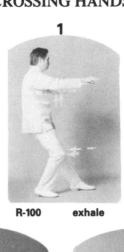

R-100   exhale

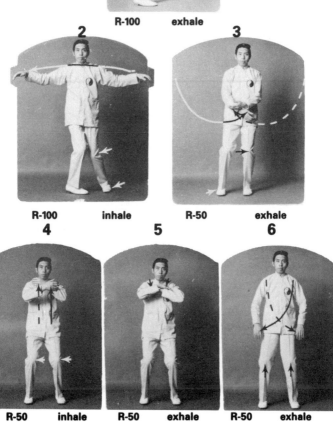

2

R-100   inhale

3

R-50   exhale

4

R-50   inhale

5

R-50   exhale

6

R-50   exhale

(60)
CROSSING HANDS

1. Shift weight back to left leg 100%.
   Move body back until arms are almost straight, palms are facing down.

2. Turn body 90° to the right.
   Move right arm across the front to the right side of the body.
   Turn left foot in on the heel 90°.

3. Shift weight to left leg 100%.
   - Move right foot back slightly until it is parallel to left foot, then shift weight back to right leg 50%.
   - Drop arms until right wrist crosses under left wrist in front of the stomach, palms are facing up.

4. Raise palms to the front of the chest, palms are facing in.

5. Turn palms inward until right wrist is on top of left wrist, palms are facing down.

6. Drop palms next to the hips, facing back.
   Stand up both legs until they are almost straight, as "Preparation" position.

(61)
PUSHING HAND

1

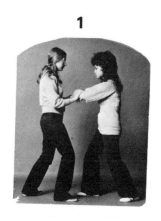

2

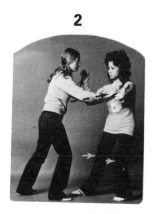

3

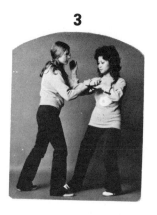

4

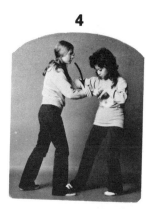

PUSHING HAND

5

6

7

8

9

10

An Incident in New York City

Some years ago in the perils of the Big Apple I was surprised by an unfortunate incident. Happily I was able to defend myself without harm. But rumors spread throughout Chinatown and both Chinese Newspapers published a story that I knocked my attacker ten feet into the air without even touching him! I tell the story now in order to dispel the idea that I possess a mystical and invisible power.

The afternoon of August 27, 1968, I became involved in a dispute with a noisy, arrogant young man disturbing the audience watching a Chinese Kung-fu movie at the Sun Sing Theater on East Broadway. Without warning, his father, a stocky, middle-aged kung-fu expert, suddenly attacked me.

At first I just blocked and neutralized his punches and pushed him away. With furious force he charged back into me. With reflex action I struck. My blow cracked his cheekbone and knocked him over five feet into the air. Falling to the ground he injured his knee. He got up and charged again. This time I broke his nose and fractured several of his ribs.

The movie Sun Sing was showing was new and exciting. Due to its popularity, quite a few martial artists packed the audience. One of the most well known, Grandmaster Peter Urban, was on the scene. He finally held back my attacker. The man had refused to stop fighting despite his serious injuries. Soon the police arrived and called an ambulance to take him to the hospital.

I don't have any mysterious force. My power resulted only from the use of my body weight in combination with speed, plus his incoming body power. This created the tremendous impact and lifting power that cracked the cheekbone and knocked him into the air. These are the fundamental principles of the Body Mechanics for the art of self-defense. The principles of my 60 movements of Tai Chi Chuan are based upon them.

"Due to numerous requests, I have decided to replace this article in this reprint of book."

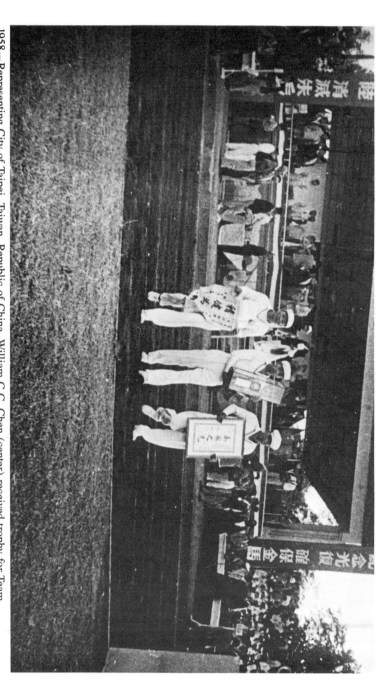

1958—Representing City of Taipei, Taiwan, Republic of China, William C.C. Chen (center) received trophy for Team Championship in the National Chinese Martial Arts Tournament of Taipei, Taiwan, R.O.C.

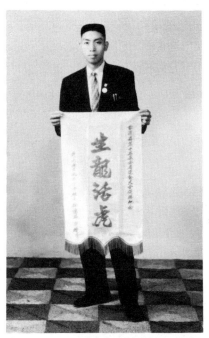

Banner Award from the 1958 National Chinese
Martial Arts Tournament. Taipei, Taiwan, R.O.C.

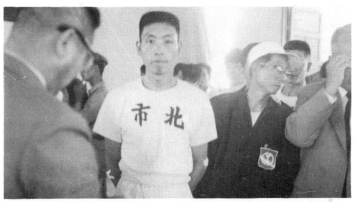

1958—Received second prize medal from the National Chinese Martial
Arts Tournament of Taipei, Taiwan, R.O.C.

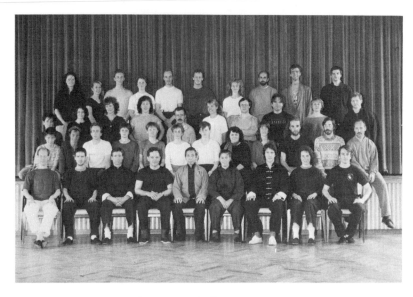

Dusseldorf, Germany
Dr. Linda Lehrhaupt

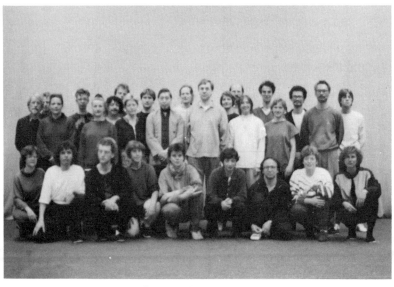

Amsterdam, Holland
Stichting Taijiquan Nederland